I0038313

Nonalcoholic Fatty Liver Disease (NAFLD)

Edited by:

Tatjana Ábel

Outpatient Department, Military Hospital Budapest, Hungary

&

Gabriella Lengyel

Semmelweis University, 2nd Department of Internal Medicine, Budapest Hungary

Nonalcoholic Fatty Liver Disease (NAFLD)

Editors: Tatjana Ábel & Gabriella Lengyel

eISBN (Online): 978-1-68108-465-7

ISBN (Print): 978-1-68108-466-4

© 2017, Bentham eBooks imprint.

Published by Bentham Science Publishers – Sharjah, UAE. All Rights Reserved.

First published in 2017.

BENTHAM SCIENCE PUBLISHERS LTD.
End User License Agreement (for non-institutional, personal use)

This is an agreement between you and Bentham Science Publishers Ltd. Please read this License Agreement carefully before using the ebook/echapter/ejournal (**"Work"**). Your use of the Work constitutes your agreement to the terms and conditions set forth in this License Agreement. If you do not agree to these terms and conditions then you should not use the Work.

Bentham Science Publishers agrees to grant you a non-exclusive, non-transferable limited license to use the Work subject to and in accordance with the following terms and conditions. This License Agreement is for non-library, personal use only. For a library / institutional / multi user license in respect of the Work, please contact: permission@benthamscience.org.

Usage Rules:

1. All rights reserved: The Work is the subject of copyright and Bentham Science Publishers either owns the Work (and the copyright in it) or is licensed to distribute the Work. You shall not copy, reproduce, modify, remove, delete, augment, add to, publish, transmit, sell, resell, create derivative works from, or in any way exploit the Work or make the Work available for others to do any of the same, in any form or by any means, in whole or in part, in each case without the prior written permission of Bentham Science Publishers, unless stated otherwise in this License Agreement.
2. You may download a copy of the Work on one occasion to one personal computer (including tablet, laptop, desktop, or other such devices). You may make one back-up copy of the Work to avoid losing it. The following DRM (Digital Rights Management) policy may also be applicable to the Work at Bentham Science Publishers' election, acting in its sole discretion:

- 25 'copy' commands can be executed every 7 days in respect of the Work. The text selected for copying cannot extend to more than a single page. Each time a text 'copy' command is executed, irrespective of whether the text selection is made from within one page or from separate pages, it will be considered as a separate / individual 'copy' command.
- 25 pages only from the Work can be printed every 7 days.

3. The unauthorised use or distribution of copyrighted or other proprietary content is illegal and could subject you to liability for substantial money damages. You will be liable for any damage resulting from your misuse of the Work or any violation of this License Agreement, including any infringement by you of copyrights or proprietary rights.

Disclaimer:

Bentham Science Publishers does not guarantee that the information in the Work is error-free, or warrant that it will meet your requirements or that access to the Work will be uninterrupted or error-free. The Work is provided "as is" without warranty of any kind, either express or implied or statutory, including, without limitation, implied warranties of merchantability and fitness for a particular purpose. The entire risk as to the results and performance of the Work is assumed by you. No responsibility is assumed by Bentham Science Publishers, its staff, editors and/or authors for any injury and/or damage to persons or property as a matter of products liability, negligence or otherwise, or from any use or operation of any methods, products instruction, advertisements or ideas contained in the Work.

Limitation of Liability:

In no event will Bentham Science Publishers, its staff, editors and/or authors, be liable for any damages, including, without limitation, special, incidental and/or consequential damages and/or damages for lost data and/or profits arising out of (whether directly or indirectly) the use or inability to use the Work. The entire liability of Bentham Science Publishers shall be limited to the amount actually paid by you for the Work.

General:

1. Any dispute or claim arising out of or in connection with this License Agreement or the Work (including non-contractual disputes or claims) will be governed by and construed in accordance with the laws of the U.A.E. as applied in the Emirate of Dubai. Each party agrees that the courts of the Emirate of Dubai shall have exclusive jurisdiction to settle any dispute or claim arising out of or in connection with this License Agreement or the Work (including non-contractual disputes or claims).

2. Your rights under this License Agreement will automatically terminate without notice and without the need for a court order if at any point you breach any terms of this License Agreement. In no event will any delay or failure by Bentham Science Publishers in enforcing your compliance with this License Agreement constitute a waiver of any of its rights.

3. You acknowledge that you have read this License Agreement, and agree to be bound by its terms and conditions. To the extent that any other terms and conditions presented on any website of Bentham Science Publishers conflict with, or are inconsistent with, the terms and conditions set out in this License Agreement, you acknowledge that the terms and conditions set out in this License Agreement shall prevail.

Bentham Science Publishers Ltd.
Executive Suite Y - 2
PO Box 7917, Saif Zone
Sharjah, U.A.E.
Email: subscriptions@benthamscience.org

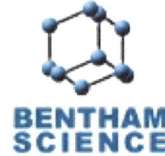

CONTENTS

FOREWORD

This book has attempted to deal with the non-alcoholic fatty liver disease (NAFLD) as well as the pathogenesis of it. Hepatocellular carcinoma (HCC) is a well-known complication of NASH, therefore, the prevention and treatment of NAFLD and its complications as early as possible have an outstanding importance. NAFLD refers to a wide spectrum of liver injury, ranging from simple steatosis to non-alcoholic steatohepatitis (NASH), advanced fibrosis and cirrhosis. NAFLD is associated with insulin resistance, type 2 diabetes mellitus.

This e-book has 9 chapters, where the diagnosis of NAFLD was detected either by imaging or histologically. They can be used to follow up the progression of the disease, monitor the efficacy of potential therapies and compare different studies.

One of the chapters deals with ultrasound (the non-invasive method), having a sensitivity of approximately 85% and specificity of 94% for the detection of moderated fatty liver. Magnetic resonance imaging (MRI) and surrogate markers Fatty Liver Index (FLI) have gained attention.

After reviewing these topics, the chapter provides a brief overview of the clinical characteristics, screening, and novel opportunities in the chemoprevention of NAFLD-related HCC. Special MRI sequences (Chemical Shift Imaging, Fast SE Imaging, elastography, spectroscopy) are capable of providing comparable results on biopsy. In contrast to biopsies, these methods provide a non-invasive way of giving a representative assessment of the whole liver. Additional therapeutic possibilities of the future may target antioxidant defense, immune–mediated mechanisms, apoptosis, and lipogenesis.

NAFLD has high prevalence in obese children, which has serious consequences without treatment.

This e-book draws the attention towards the fact that early intervention is most important when NAFLD is diagnosed, which should include early lifestyle modification (nutrition and physical activity, avoidance of smoking).

I feel that the students and medical doctors should have some Knowledge of these important concepts. I believe this is necessary in view of the importance of this system in clinical medicine.

Erzsébet Fehér
Semmelweis University
Budapest, Hungary

PREFACE

Non-alcoholic fatty liver disease (NAFLD) is one of the most common causes of elevated liver enzymes and chronic liver disease in Western countries. Patients with elevated liver enzymes in the absence of alcohol consumption and secondary causes of liver disease are described as having NAFLD, which is an independent predictor of future risk of cardiovascular diseases, type 2 diabetes and metabolic syndrome (hypertension, abdominal obesity, dyslipidemia, glucose intolerance). The 'two hit' theory introduced in 1998 by Day and James proposes that development of NASH requires a second hit to an already sensitized liver by steatosis which constitutes the first hit. Recently, the 'two hit' theory was strongly challenged and 'one-hit' and 'multiple-hit' theories have been proposed. Insulin resistance and obesity are two important factors of pathogenesis of NAFLD. The pathomechanism of NAFLD involves multiple genetic and environmental factors. Besides the genetic susceptibility to develop the disease, it appears that promoting factors notably include: lipid intermediate accumulation, altered expression of pro-inflammatory cytokines and mitochondrial dysfunction.

Tatjana Ábel
Outpatient Department, Military Hospital,
Budapest
Hungary

&

Gabriella Lengyel
Semmelweis University, 2nd Department of Internal Medicine,
Budapest
Hungary

List of Contributors

Alajos Pár	First Department of Medicine, University of Pécs, Pécs, Hungary
Gabriella Lengyel	Semmelweis University, 2nd Department of Internal Medicine, Budapest, Hungary
Gabriella Par	First Department of Medicine, University of Pécs, Pécs, Hungary
György Baffy	VA Boston Healthcare System and Brigham and Women's Hospital, Harvard Medical School, Boston, Massachusetts, United States of America
István Tornai	University of Debrecen, Clinical Center, Department of Medicine, Division of Gastroenterology, Debrecen, Hungary
Krisztina Hagymási	Semmelweis University, 2nd Department of Internal Medicine, Budapest, Hungary
Omar Giyab	University of Pécs, Medical School, Department of Radiology, Pécs, Pécs, Hungary
Peter Nagy	Department of Pathology and Experimental Cancer Research, Semmelweis University, Budapest, Hungary
Tatjana Ábel	Outpatient Department, Military Hospital, Budapest, Hungary. Faculty of Health Sciences, Semmelweis University, Budapest, Hungary
Zoltán Harmat	University of Pécs, Medical School, Department of Radiology, Pécs, Pécs, Hungary
Zsuzsanna Almássy	Department of Toxicology and Metabolic Diseases, Heim Pál Children's Hospital, Budapest, Hungary

Nonalcoholic Fatty Liver Disease (NAFLD)

Nonalcoholic Fatty Liver Disease (NAFLD)

CHAPTER 1

Epidemiology of NAFLD

Alajos Par[*]

First Department of Medicine, University of Pécs, Hungary

Abstract: Non-alcoholic fatty liver disease (NAFLD) refers to a wide spectrum of liver injuries, ranging from simple steatosis to non-alcoholic steatohepatitis (NASH), advanced fibrosis and cirrhosis. NAFLD is associated with insulin resistance, type 2 diabetes mellitus, obesity, hypertriglyceridemia and hypertension; thus, it is regarded as a hepatic component of the metabolic syndrome, and an independent risk factor for cardiovascular disease.

NAFLD and NASH are common causes of chronic liver disease and elevated liver enzymes. Their worldwide prevalence continues to increase with the growing obesity epidemic. Understanding the epidemiology of these pathologies is essential for developing treatment and prevention strategies. The prevalence of NAFLD and NASH in the general population has been assessed with a variety of diagnostic means, such as liver biopsy, non-invasive radiological and ultrasonic techniques, elevated liver enzymes and combinations of clinical variables. Because liver biopsy is not appropriate for population studies, only on the basis of autopsy studies it has been suggested that 3-5% of individuals in the general population might have NASH, and 20-30% of people in industrialized countries have NAFLD. The prevalence of NAFLD increases with age, it is highest in males between 40-65 years and is higher in Hispanics and lower in African-Americans.

Ultrasound is the non-invasive method most commonly used to assess NAFLD, having a sensitivity of approximately 85% and a specificity of 94% for the detection of moderated fatty liver. *Magnetic resonance imaging (MRI)* has also been used to perform population studies, but it is less portable and more expensive than US. Among *surrogate markers Fatty Liver Index* (FLI) has gained much attention.

Several studies have shown that NASH is a risk factor for liver fibrosis. At the same time, most cases of fatty liver and even fibrosis can regress, particularly due to life style modification and weight loss. Based on the well-established strong association of the NAFLD with the metabolic syndrome and the epidemic of obesity, the prevalence of NASH is expected to increase in the next decade, leading to cirrhosis and even HCC. There is a need to perform larger, longitudinal studies that assess the long-term natural

[*] **Corresponding author Alajos Par:** First Department of Medicine, University of Pécs, Hungary; Tel: +36 72 536 000; Fax: +36 72 536 148; E-mail: par.alajos@pte.hu

Tatjana Ábel & Gabriella Lengyel (Eds.)
All rights reserved-© 2017 Bentham Science Publishers

history of NAFLD with validated non-invasive biomarkers and by integrating morbidity and mortality data.

Keywords: Epidemiology, Natural history, Non-alcoholic fatty liver disease, Non-alcoholic steatohepatitis, Prevalence, Risk factors.

INTRODUCTION

Over the past 5 years several comprehensive reviews studied the epidemiology and natural history of non-alcoholic fatty liver disease (NAFLD) and non-alcoholic steatohepatitis (NASH). Among them, *Byrne et al.* [1] when discussing the metabolic disturbances in NAFLD, emphasized that since obesity and diabetes are increasing in prevalence worldwide, there is a marked increase in NAFLD, which occurs in individuals of all ages and ethnic groups, and at the same time, it is an independent risk factor for cardiovascular disease (CVD). *Cheung* and *Sanyal* also underlined that NAFLD is the most common cause of chronic liver disease in North America and some Western countries associated with the metabolic syndrome, and its prevalence is estimated to be as high as 35% in some populations linked to the growing epidemic of obesity [2]. *Ratziu et al.,* based on the EASL 2009 special conference, outlined the concepts on NAFLD, as an increasingly relevant public health issue. Since recently NAFLD is a frequent condition, it often co-exists with other chronic liver diseases, such as alcohol abuse, and HCV infection or hemochromatosis, EASL suggested a shift in diagnostic concept of NAFLD from a "negative" diagnosis of exclusion (to drop the "negative" definition of "nonalcoholic") to a positive one, based on the presence of an underlying condition, instead of the absence of an unrelated disease. Thus, according to EASL, there would be a need for a change in nomenclature, discarding the negative definition, and using a name of *"metabolic steatosis or metabolic steatohepatitis"* [3]. In their overview, *Lewis* and *Mohanty* pointed out that NAFLD affects approximately 20-30% of population in industrialized countries, males and females are both equally affected; however, some studies revealed that it is more common in men than women in morbidly obese and Asian populations [4]. In 2011, *Vernon et al.* in a paper summarized the epidemiology and natural history of NAFLD based on clinical literature published over the past 30 years. They emphasized that understanding the epidemiology of NAFLD is essential for developing effective treatment and prevention strategies, which is of pivotal importance, because the prevalence of NAFLD and NASH is expected to increase in the next decade, leading to advanced fibrosis, cirrhosis and even HCC [5]. *Bhatia et al.* [6] provided a state-of-art article of the evidence linking NAFLD with CVD, the potential mechanisms underlying this association, its relation to insulin resistance and the metabolic syndrome, in the context of increased CV risk. The role of NASH as a potential independent CV risk factor has gained considerable importance such as an awareness of this disease is essential for practicing cardiologists, given that it affects 20-30% of general population. *Weiß et al.* [7] when reviewing the publications on NAFLD that appeared between 1995 and 2013 stated that at present some 5% to 20% of patients with NAFLD develop NASH, and fewer than 5% of cases progress to cirrhosis. Approximately 0.05% to 0.3% may be the prevalence of cirrhosis in the general population and 2% of cirrhotic patients per year develop HCC. Recently *Bedogni et al.* provided a concise overview of the epidemiology of NAFLD published between January 2011 and October 2013; they noted, that NAFLD may be a separate entity, rather than an additional component of metabolic syndrome, but it remains to be tested, whether metabolic syndrome and NAFLD contribute to "hard outcomes" in the general population independently [8].

PREVALENCE OF NAFLD AND NASH

The prevalence of NAFLD and NASH in general population depends on the diagnostic methods, such as liver biopsy, radiological and ultrasonic techniques, elevated liver enzymes, and combination of clinical variables.

Liver Biopsy and Autopsy Studies

Liver biopsy (LB) has long been regarded as gold standard for the diagnosis and staging of NAFLD and NASH, though it is an invasive measure and cannot be used in population-based studies. Yet, valuable findings have been reported for liver **transplant donors** who are considered healthy people. A Korean study in which LB-s were performed on 589 consecutive potential liver transplant donors reported NAFLD prevalence of 51% [9].

In the USA 20% of donors were ineligible for donation based on the degree of steatosis (>30%) [10]. A high prevalence of histological NAFLD has been described in healthy living liver donors: 12-18% in Europe [11, 12], and 27-38% in the USA [13, 14]. In healthy living liver donors, the prevalence of NASH ranges from 3% to 16% in Europe [11, 12], and from 6% to 15% in the USA [13, 14].

The results of **autopsy** series showed mixed data regarding the prevalence of NAFLD. In an autopsy series of lean individuals from Canada, the prevalence of NASH and fibrosis was 3% and 7%, respectively [15], while a study from Greece showed evidence of steatosis in 31% and NASH in 40% of autopsied cases of ischemic heart disease or traffic accident death after exclusion of HBV positivity or known liver disease [16]. Furthermore, the studies using current histological definition, have shown a high prevalence of NASH among steatosis cases: 43-55% in patients with increased aminotransferases [17], and 49% in morbidly obese patients [18, 19]. On the basis of autopsy studies it has been suggested, that 3-5% of individuals in the general population might have NASH [20, 21].

Ultrasound (US)

US as a non-invasive method is the technique most commonly used to assess NAFLD in the general population. Although, it may have a sensitivity of 84.8% and specificity of 93.6% for the detection of moderated fatty liver [20, 22], US is unable to diagnose steatosis when it is less than 20-30% on liver biopsy, thus the prevalence of NAFLD may be underestimated by this means. Yet, most general population studies are based on US studies. The prevalence of NAFLD in the general population is assessed by US is 20-30% in Europe [23], as well as in the Middle East [24], and 15% in the Far East [25].

Armstrong et al. [26] studying NAFLD in a large, primary care practice in the UK, identified 1118 asymptomatic individuals with increased liver function tests, and established NAFLD in 25% of subjects. In a multicentric population study from Spain, the prevalence of NAFLD by US was 33% in men and 20% in women [27].

In a study performed in middle-aged USA Army personnel seeking medical care for unspecified medical condition, the prevalence of US-defined and histo-logically confirmed fatty liver was 48% [28].

Over 10 to 12 years, the prevalence of NAFLD identified by US in 35 519 Japanese individuals increased from 13% to 30% [29].

Magnetic Resonance Imaging (MRI)

MRI has also been used to perform population studies, but is less portable and much more expensive than US [20, 30]. MRI identified NAFLD in 31% of multi-ethnic, population based samples from the USA [28].

Non-invasive Biomarker for Fibrosis: Fibrotest

When screening the general population with a noninvasive biomarker **Fibrotest**, for fibrosis, *Poynard et al.* found a prevalence of advanced fibrosis of 3% [31]. It is estimated that 25% of the adult Western population have NAFLD and only half of them have elevated liver function tests, and between 1% and 2% of the general population might have advanced fibrosis due to NASH [32].

Elevation in Liver Enzymes and Combinations of Clinical Variables

Alanine aminotransferase (ALT) and aspartate aminotransferase (AST) as non-invasive indicators, showed the prevalence of NAFLD ranging from 3% to 21% in population studies [33, 34]. Although elevated ALT is generally associated with histological NASH, several patients with normal ALT may also have NASH and even advanced fibrosis. Thus, ALT activity alone cannot be used to rule out significant liver disease in patients suspected of having NAFLD and NASH [35].

Two *combinations* of clinical variables for NAFLD epidemiology studies are Fatty liver Index, **FLI** (BMI, waist circumference, triglyceride and GGT) [36 - 39], and Lipid Accumulation Product, **LAP** (waist circumference and fasting triglyceride) [40]. These indices may contribute to epidemiological studies.

Taken together, now it is widely accepted that 20-30% of individuals in Western world have NAFLD and similar figures are being provided for Eastern countries as well. NAFLD has become the most commonly US-diagnosed cause of chronic liver disease, partially in connection with the epidemic of obesity as well as with the greater awareness of the disease. Worldwide, the assumed prevalence of NAFLD is between 6% and 33%, with a median of 20%, while the prevalence of NASH is 3% to 5% [3, 5, 41, 42].

RISK FACTORS

Vernon et al. studying the **risk factors** of NAFLD have pointed out that age, gender, race and ethnicity as well as the metabolic alterations, all play a significant role in the development of the disease [5].

Age

The prevalence of NAFLD increases with age [43 - 47], and it is highest in males between 40 and 65 years [14]. *Frith et al.* showed an association between the prevalence of NAFLD and fibrosis with age; they found that older patients had higher grades of fibrosis, and cirrhotic patients were older than non-cirrhotic patients [48]. Another study performed in a cohort of octogenarians reported a prevalence rate of 46% [43].

Cryptogenic cirrhosis, (which is considered "burned-out NASH") was found to be more common in older diabetic patients with current or past obesity [49]. Older age increases the risk of developing fibrosis, cirrhosis and hepatocellular carcinoma (HCC) as well as type 2 diabetes mellitus [50]. It seems that the association between age and the high prevalence of NASH as well as the higher stage of fibrosis in NAFLD may be related to the duration of disease rather than to age itself [5].

Gender

NASH was initially thought to be more common in women, and a few studies suggested that female gender is associated with NAFLD and fibrosis [51, 52]. On the other hand, some studies revealed that NAFLD is more common in men than women in morbidly obese and Asian populations [53, 54]. It is possible that NAFLD behaves differently in men and women, but the reason is not known yet.

Race, Ethnicity and Gene Variants

Prevalence of NAFLD differs with **race and ethnicity**. While Hispanics have the highest frequency of NAFLD, followed by non-Hispanic Whites, with the lowest rate reported in African-Americans [28, 55 - 57]. The prevalence of NAFLD in American Indian and Alaska-Native populations ranges from 0.4% to 2% [58]. The rising incidence of NAFLD in several Asian countries including China, Korea, Japan and India was reported. Asian patients with NAFLD display higher levels of visceral adiposity at lower body mass index than the Caucasian population [59]. Central obesity is associated with insulin resistance and may be a more important risk factor in Asian population than in Caucasian population [60]. The explanation for ethnic differences in the prevalence is not clear; it is possible that NAFLD may be affected by yet unidentified genetic and environmental factors.

Earlier *Browning et al.* [55] reported that these differences may be attributable to biologic differences rather than lower rate of insulin resistance. Since African-American (AA) individuals were less likely to develop steatosis than White and Hispanic subjects, it seemed that inherent biological differences, *e.g.* lower rates of hypertriglyceridemia and low density lipoprotein cholesterol levels among AA subjects might have contributed to this lower incidence of steatosis in AA population.

Family members of subjects with NAFLS are also at increased risk. The observed familiar clustering on NADFLD suggests the role of genetic factors. Some studies of family-based cohorts indicate that the heritability of steatosis is approximately 27% [61, 62].

According to the genom-wide associate studies, the most important genetic factor to NAFLD seems to be the I148M allele of the PNPLA3 gene, which encodes *adiponutrin* [63 - 65]. This allele is prevalent in Hispanics (49%), the group most susceptible to NAFLD, while lower frequencies were found in Caucasians (23%) and African Americans (17%). NASH occurred with higher prevalence in I148M homozygotes (OR 3.488) [66].

Metabolic Disorders

It is well known, that NAFLD is more prevalent in patients with metabolic alterations such as type 2 diabetes mellitus, obesity, hypertriglyceridemia than the general population. A study of patients with type 2 diabetes mellitus reported a 69% prevalence of ultrasonographic NAFLD. Similarly, the prevalence of NASH increases in parallel with components of metabolic syndrome [67 - 69]. Longitudinal studies revealed a chronological association between the progression of the metabolic syndrome and the occurrence of NAFLD [70].

In the USA, the proportion of NAFLD among patients with chronic liver disease rose from 47% to 75%, over a twenty-year period, between 1988 and 2008, due to the increase in metabolic diseases and the aging population. At the same time, the prevalence of obesity rose from 21% to 33%, type 2 diabetes mellitus from 5.6% to 9.1%, and insulin resistance from 23% to 35% [71, 72].

The frequency of simple steatosis in *obese* individuals ranges from 30% to 37% and NAFLD ranges from 57% of overweight individuals to 98% of nondiabetic obese patients. The prevalence of NAFLD and cirrhosis in a cohort of obese patients undergoing intraoperative liver biopsy and gastric bypass was 63% and 2%, respectively [73]. Others showed that over 95% of bariatric surgery patients had fatty liver, 20-30% has NASH and 10 have advanced fibrosis. The median prevalence of NASH in the obese population is 33% ranging from 10 to 56% [74, 75].

Smits et al. suggested that NAFLD may be a separate entity, rather than an additional component of metabolic syndrome [76], but it remains to be tested, whether MS and NAFLD contribute to "hard outcomes" in the general population independently [8].

Polycystic Ovarian Syndrome (PCOS)

Interestingly, polycystic ovarian syndrome (PCOS) was proposed as the ovarian manifestation of metabolic syndrome as 41-55% of PCOS women had concomitant NAFLD, while in the non-PCOS control group the incidence of

NAFLD was 19% [77, 78]. Thus, PCOS patients may be at risk for developing NAFLD and NASH [5]. Many potential links between PCOS and NAFLD have been proposed, most notably insulin resistance and hyperandrogenemia. Further studies are needed to clarify the association between PCOS and NAFLD.

Hepatitis C Virus (HCV)

HCV infection may also be a risk factor for NAFLD. It was shown that HCV exacerbates metabolic syndrome, increasing insulin resistance [79]. Steatosis is present in approximately 50% of patients with chronic hepatitis C, especially often in association with HCV genotype 3 infection [79, 80].

NATURAL HISTORY

Regarding the long-term outcomes and in terms of potential for progression, NAFLD patients fall into two categories: *NASH* and *non-NASH*. The non-NASH subtype includes all individuals with *simple steatosis*, which does not progress or progresses very slowly [81]; on the other hand, NASH patients at diagnosis showed inflammation and even bridging fibrosis in 25-33% including cirrhosis in 10-15% [82].

Harrison et al. reported that based on paired liver biopsies, 32% of NASH patients showed progressing fibrosis over a median follow-up of 5.7 years [83]. Similarly, a repeat biopsy study showed that 53% of NASH patients had fibrosis progression by at least one stage after a median time of 6.4 years [52].

Independent predictors of *fibrosis* are mainly age (>45 years), diabetes, BMI (>28 kg/m^2), hypertension, and degree of IR [84]. The strongest predictor of progression is necro-inflammation on the initial biopsy. End-stage NASH is a cause of *cryptogenic cirrhosis*, mainly because steatosis and liver cell injury can disappear at this stage. Approximately 30-75% of cryptogenic cirrhosis can be attributed to "burned-out" NASH [49].

Liver failure is often the first presentation of NASH cirrhosis, and occurs after 7-10 years in 38-45% of cirrhotic patients [85]. Obese and diabetic patients have an increased risk of hepatocellular carcinoma (HCC) [86]. While simple steatosis does not increase overall or liver-related mortality, NASH increases overall mortality by 35-85% compared to general population and cardiovascular mortality is increased twofold in NASH patients [87]. Liver related mortality is increased 9-10 fold with NASH cirrhosis [88].

According to *Adams et al.* [89] in a community-based report of NAFLD patients from the U.S.A, mortality rate was 13% after a mean follow-up of 7.6 years. When *Rafiq et al.* [90] assessed the mortality in biopsy proven NAFLD patients after 8 years follow-up, liver related mortality developed in 11% of NASH patients compared to 2% of the non-NASH patients. *Ekstedt et al.* found increased mortality in NASH after 13.7 years of follow-up, but not in patients with simple steatosis [87]. Furthermore, it was also shown that the lifestyle modification and weight loss, as well as the bariatric intervention (gastric bypass) may lead to the resolution of steatosis. Already 4% body weight loss can result in significant decrease in steatosis in 56% of patients [91]. An earlier study of 90 biopsied bariatric patients showed that 18% had the same degree of steatosis, histologically improved 28%, and 54% had normal histology by the second biopsy [92].

Bedogni et al. [8] and *Kim et al.* [93] also emphasized that while studies have shown that NASH is a risk factor for liver fibrosis, cirrhosis and HCC; at the same time, even fibrosis can regress. Serial biopsy studies demonstrated that fibrosis in NAFLD patients might improve. *Wong et al.* [81] found that 27% NAFLD patients had fibrosis progression, 48% had static disease, and 25% had fibrosis regression after 3 years of the initial diagnosis.

Taking these studies into consideration, based on histology data suggest that only patients with NASH show the progressive form of the NAFLD; in addition, insulin resistance, type 2 diabetes mellitus or other components of metabolic syndrome are risk factors for developing advanced liver injury. As patients with cryptogenic cirrhosis are, on average, 10 years older than patients with NASH, it is conceivable, that in patients with cirrhosis the disease started with NASH and on over a decade it progressed to cirrhosis.

Although NAFLD is mainly associated with obesity (*e.g.* with prevalence of 28%), it can be found even *in lean individuals* (BMI <25 kg/m^2): a prevalence of 7% NAFLD was observed in such cases, characterized by younger age, higher insulin sensitivity and lower frequency of metabolic syndrome [26].

Finally, the association between NASH and **hepatocellular carcinoma** (HCC) may provide another type of indirect evidence supporting of the progressive nature of NASH [94]. *Hashimoto et al.* [50] found that with a median follow-up of 40.3 months the 5-year cumulative incidence of HCC was 8% among patients with NASH and advanced fibrosis. *Bugianesi et al.* showed a 7% overall prevalence of HCC in cryptogenic cirrhosis [95]. A multivariate analysis revealed that hypertriglyceridemia and type 2 diabetes mellitus are associated with cryptogenic cirrhosis and HCC. In another study, 91% of NASH related HCC patients were obese or had type 2 diabetes mellitus or dyslipidemia, suggesting that these risk factors may be involved in the pathogenesis of NASH related HCC [96].

BRIEFLY ON NAFLD AND CARDIOVASCULAR DISEASE (CVD)

Targher et al. [97] emphasized that the role of NAFLD as a potential CV risk factor is of considerable importance, and an awareness of this disease is essential for practicing cardiologists, given that it affects 20-30% of general population. Up to now, several studies reported an increased incidence of adverse cardiovascular (CV) events in NAFLD patients compared with the general population [98 - 103]. A significant association between increased gamma-glutamyl transferase (GGT) values and CVD mortality has been shown over a median of 12-year follow-up [100]. A meta-analysis of 10 studies also confirmed the independent association between elevated GGT and CV events [101]. Yet, alanine aminotransferase (ALT) has been reported to be more closely related to liver fat content than GGT [14], and population-based examinations have shown an independent association between ALT and CVD mortality [102]. The correlation of elevated ALT and GGT with CV disease reflected their significant associations with insulin resistance, which is itself a risk factor for CVD. Using US as a diagnostic tool for NAFLD, large, community-based studies also documented an independent association with CV disease [103]. *Hamaguchi et al.* performing a prospective analysis of 1637 healthy subjects found 19% NAFLD by US. After a 5-year follow-up, 5.2% of the NAFLD patients suffered from CV event compared with 1.0% of the non-NAFLD group [98]. Smaller long-term prospective studies in biopsy-proven NAFLD showed higher mortality rates compared with a matched reference population. Only patients with NASH rather than simple steatosis had significantly reduced survival [17, 87].

SUMMARY

NAFLD is present in 20-30% of general populations of industrialized countries and is the most prevalent chronic liver disease, often associated with obesity and diabetes mellitus. Among NAFLD patients, NASH occurs in 10-20%, thus the prevalence of NASH in the population is approximately is 2-5%. NASH accounts for more than 50% cryptogenic cirrhosis which may progress to hepatocellular carcinoma (HCC). Due to the dramatic increase in overweight in the industrialized world, there is a similar increase in the prevalence of NAFLD and NASH. Today more than 80% of NAFLD or NASH patients show hyperlipidemia, 50% have insulin resistance, 40% are obese and 20-30% have type 2 diabetes mellitus, *i.e.* there is a strong association between NAFLD and metabolic syndrome. Hypertriglyceridemia and diabetes are associated with cryptogenic cirrhosis. Since approximately 90% of NASH related HCC patients are obese or have type 2 diabetes mellitus or dyslipidemia, it can be assumed that these risk factors may be involved in the pathogenesis of NASH related HCC. Several studies reported an increased incidence of adverse cardiovascular events in NAFLD patients compared with the general population. Prospective studies in biopsy-proven NAFLD showed higher mortality rates compared with a matched reference population, but only patients with NASH rather than simple steatosis had significantly reduced survival.

CONFLICT OF INTEREST

The author confirms that he has no conflict of interest to declare for this publication.

ACKNOWLEDGEMENTS

Declared none.

REFERENCES

[1] Byrne CD, Olufadi R, Bruce KD, Cagampang FR, Ahmed MH. Metabolic disturbances in non-alcoholic fatty liver disease. Clin Sci 2009; 116(7): 539-64.
[http://dx.doi.org/10.1042/CS20080253] [PMID: 19243311]

[2] Cheung O, Sanyal AJ. Recent advances in nonalcoholic fatty liver disease. Curr Opin Gastroenterol 2010; 26(3): 202-8.
[http://dx.doi.org/10.1097/MOG.0b013e328337b0c4] [PMID: 20168226]

[3] Ratziu V, Bellentani S, Cortez-Pinto H, Day C, Marchesini G. A position statement on NAFLD/NASH based on the EASL 2009 special conference. J Hepatol 2010; 53(2): 372-84.
[http://dx.doi.org/10.1016/j.jhep.2010.04.008] [PMID: 20494470]

[4] Lewis JR, Mohanty SR. Nonalcoholic fatty liver disease: a review and update. Dig Dis Sci 2010; 55(3): 560-78.
[http://dx.doi.org/10.1007/s10620-009-1081-0] [PMID: 20101463]

[5] Vernon G, Baranova A, Younossi ZM. Systematic review: the epidemiology and natural history of non-alcoholic fatty liver disease and non-alcoholic steatohepatitis in adults. Aliment Pharmacol Ther 2011; 34(3): 274-85.
[http://dx.doi.org/10.1111/j.1365-2036.2011.04724.x] [PMID: 21623852]

[6] Bhatia LS, Curzen NP, Calder PC, Byrne CD. Non-alcoholic fatty liver disease: a new and important cardiovascular risk factor? Eur Heart J 2012; 33(10): 1190-200.
[http://dx.doi.org/10.1093/eurheartj/ehr453] [PMID: 22408036]

[7] Weiß J, Rau M, Geier A. Non-alcoholic fatty liver disease: epidemiology, clinical course, investigation, and treatment. Dtsch Arztebl Int 2014; 111(26): 447-52.
[PMID: 25019921]

[8] Bedogni G, Nobili V, Tiribelli C. Epidemiology of fatty liver: an update. World J Gastroenterol 2014; 20(27): 9050-4.

[9]   Lee JY, Kim KM, Lee SG, *et al.* Prevalence and risk factors of non-alcoholic fatty liver disease in potential living liver donors in Korea: a review of 589 consecutive liver biopsies in a single center. J Hepatol 2007; 47(2): 239-44.
[http://dx.doi.org/10.1016/j.jhep.2007.02.007] [PMID: 17400323]

[10]   Marcos A, Fisher RA, Ham JM, *et al.* Selection and outcome of living donors for adult to adult right lobe transplantation. Transplantation 2000; 69(11): 2410-5.
[http://dx.doi.org/10.1097/00007890-200006150-00034] [PMID: 10868650]

[11]   Minervini MI, Ruppert K, Fontes P, *et al.* Liver biopsy findings from healthy potential living liver donors: reasons for disqualification, silent diseases and correlation with liver injury tests. J Hepatol 2009; 50(3): 501-10.
[http://dx.doi.org/10.1016/j.jhep.2008.10.030] [PMID: 19155086]

[12]   Nadalin S, Malagó M, Valentin-Gamazo C, *et al.* Preoperative donor liver biopsy for adult living donor liver transplantation: risks and benefits. Liver Transpl 2005; 11(8): 980-6.
[http://dx.doi.org/10.1002/lt.20462] [PMID: 16035060]

[13]   Ryan CK, Johnson LA, Germin BI, Marcos A. One hundred consecutive hepatic biopsies in the workup of living donors for right lobe liver transplantation. Liver Transpl 2002; 8(12): 1114-22.
[http://dx.doi.org/10.1053/jlts.2002.36740] [PMID: 12474149]

[14]   Tran TT, Changsri C, Shackleton CR, *et al.* Living donor liver transplantation: histological abnormalities found on liver biopsies of apparently healthy potential donors. J Gastroenterol Hepatol 2006; 21(2): 381-3.
[http://dx.doi.org/10.1111/j.1440-1746.2005.03968.x] [PMID: 16509862]

[15]   Wanless IR, Lentz JS. Fatty liver hepatitis (steatohepatitis) and obesity: an autopsy study with analysis of risk factors. Hepatology 1990; 12(5): 1106-10.
[http://dx.doi.org/10.1002/hep.1840120505] [PMID: 2227807]

[16]   Zois CD, Baltayiannis GH, Bekiari A, *et al.* Steatosis and steatohepatitis in postmortem material from Northwestern Greece. World J Gastroenterol 2010; 16(31): 3944-9.
[http://dx.doi.org/10.3748/wjg.v16.i31.3944] [PMID: 20712056]

[17]   Söderberg C, Stål P, Askling J, *et al.* Decreased survival of subjects with elevated liver function tests during a 28-year follow-up. Hepatology 2010; 51(2): 595-602.
[http://dx.doi.org/10.1002/hep.23314] [PMID: 20014114]

[18]   Campos GM, Bambha K, Vittinghoff E, *et al.* A clinical scoring system for predicting nonalcoholic steatohepatitis in morbidly obese patients. Hepatology 2008; 47(6): 1916-23.
[http://dx.doi.org/10.1002/hep.22241] [PMID: 18433022]

[19]   Machado M, Marques-Vidal P, Cortez-Pinto H. Hepatic histology in obese patients undergoing bariatric surgery. J Hepatol 2006; 45(4): 600-6.
[http://dx.doi.org/10.1016/j.jhep.2006.06.013] [PMID: 16899321]

[20]   Festi D, Schiumerini R, Marzi L, *et al.* Review article: the diagnosis of non-alcoholic fatty liver disease availability and accuracy of non-invasive methods. Aliment Pharmacol Ther 2013; 37(4): 392-400.
[http://dx.doi.org/10.1111/apt.12186] [PMID: 23278163]

[21]   Scaglioni F, Ciccia S, Marino M, Bedogni G, Bellentani S. ASH and NASH. Dig Dis 2011; 29(2): 202-10.
[http://dx.doi.org/10.1159/000323886] [PMID: 21734385]

[22]   Hernaez R, Lazo M, Bonekamp S, *et al.* Diagnostic accuracy and reliability of ultrasonography for the detection of fatty liver: a meta-analysis. Hepatology 2011; 54(3): 1082-90.
[http://dx.doi.org/10.1002/hep.24452] [PMID: 21618575]

[23]   Bedogni G, Miglioli L, Masutti F, Tiribelli C, Marchesini G, Bellentani S. Prevalence of and risk factors for nonalcoholic fatty liver disease: the Dionysos nutrition and liver study. Hepatology 2005; 42(1): 44-52.
[http://dx.doi.org/10.1002/hep.20734] [PMID: 15895401]

[24]   Zelber-Sagi S, Nitzan-Kaluski D, Halpern Z, Oren R. Prevalence of primary non-alcoholic fatty liver disease in a population-based study and its association with biochemical and anthropometric measures. Liver Int 2006; 26(7): 856-63.
[http://dx.doi.org/10.1111/j.1478-3231.2006.01311.x] [PMID: 16911469]

[25]   Fan JG, Zhu J, Li XJ, *et al.* Prevalence of and risk factors for fatty liver in a general population of Shanghai, China. J Hepatol 2005; 43(3): 508-14.
[http://dx.doi.org/10.1016/j.jhep.2005.02.042] [PMID: 16006003]

[26]   Armstrong MJ, Houlihan DD, Bentham L, *et al.* Presence and severity of non-alcoholic fatty liver disease in a large prospective primary care cohort. J Hepatol 2012; 56(1): 234-40.
[http://dx.doi.org/10.1016/j.jhep.2011.03.020] [PMID: 21703178]

[26]   Caballería L, Pera G, Auladell MA, *et al.* Prevalence and factors associated with the presence of nonalcoholic fatty liver disease in an adult population in Spain. Eur J Gastroenterol Hepatol 2010; 22(1): 24-32.
[http://dx.doi.org/10.1097/MEG.0b013e32832fcdf0] [PMID: 19730384]

[28]   Williams CD, Stengel J, Asike MI, *et al.* Prevalence of nonalcoholic fatty liver disease and nonalcoholic steatohepatitis among a largely middle-aged population utilizing ultrasound and liver biopsy: a prospective study. Gastroenterology 2011; 140(1): 124-31.
[http://dx.doi.org/10.1053/j.gastro.2010.09.038] [PMID: 20858492]

[29]   Kojima S, Watanabe N, Numata M, Ogawa T, Matsuzaki S. Increase in the prevalence of fatty liver in Japan over the past 12 years: analysis of clinical background. J Gastroenterol 2003; 38(10): 954-61.
[http://dx.doi.org/10.1007/s00535-003-1178-8] [PMID: 14614602]

[30]   Bedogni G, Miglioli L, Masutti F, *et al.* Incidence and natural course of fatty liver in the general population: the Dionysos study. Hepatology 2007; 46(5): 1387-91.
[http://dx.doi.org/10.1002/hep.21827] [PMID: 17685472]

[31]   Poynard T, Lebray P, Ingiliz P, *et al.* Prevalence of liver fibrosis and risk factors in a general population using non-invasive biomarkers (FibroTest). BMC Gastroenterol 2010; 10: 40.
[http://dx.doi.org/10.1186/1471-230X-10-40] [PMID: 20412588]

[32]   Ratziu V, Voiculescu M, Poynard T. Touching some firm ground in the epidemiology of NASH. J Hepatol 2012; 56(1): 23-5. [Editorial].
[http://dx.doi.org/10.1016/j.jhep.2011.08.002] [PMID: 21875499]

[33]   Clark JM, Brancati FL, Diehl AM. The prevalence and etiology of elevated aminotransferase levels in the United States. Am J Gastroenterol 2003; 98(5): 960-7.
[http://dx.doi.org/10.1111/j.1572-0241.2003.07486.x] [PMID: 12809815]

[34]   Ioannou GN, Boyko EJ, Lee SP. The prevalence and predictors of elevated serum aminotransferase activity in the United States in 19992002. Am J Gastroenterol 2006; 101(1): 76-82.
[http://dx.doi.org/10.1111/j.1572-0241.2005.00341.x] [PMID: 16405537]

[35]   Amarapurkar DN, Patel ND. Clinical spectrum and natural history of non-alcoholic steatohepatitis with normal alanine aminotransferase values. Trop Gastroenterol 2004; 25(3): 130-4.
[PMID: 15682660]

[36]   Bedogni G, Bellentani S, Miglioli L, *et al.* The Fatty Liver Index: a simple and accurate predictor of hepatic steatosis in the general population. BMC Gastroenterol 2006; 6: 33.
[http://dx.doi.org/10.1186/1471-230X-6-33] [PMID: 17081293]

[37] Jung CH, Lee WJ, Hwang JY, *et al.* Assessment of the fatty liver index as an indicator of hepatic steatosis for predicting incident diabetes independently of insulin resistance in a Korean population. Diabet Med 2013; 30(4): 428-35.
[http://dx.doi.org/10.1111/dme.12104] [PMID: 23278318]

[38] Kozakova M, Palombo C, Eng MP, *et al.* Fatty liver index, gamma-glutamyltransferase, and early carotid plaques. Hepatology 2012; 55(5): 1406-15.
[http://dx.doi.org/10.1002/hep.25555] [PMID: 22334565]

[39] Koehler EM, Schouten JN, Hansen BE, Hofman A, Stricker BH, Janssen HL. External validation of the fatty liver index for identifying nonalcoholic fatty liver disease in a population-based study. Clin Gastroenterol Hepatol 2013; 11(9): 1201-4.
[http://dx.doi.org/10.1016/j.cgh.2012.12.031] [PMID: 23353640]

[40] Bedogni G, Kahn HS, Bellentani S, Tiribelli C. A simple index of lipid overaccumulation is a good marker of liver steatosis. BMC Gastroenterol 2010; 10: 98.
[http://dx.doi.org/10.1186/1471-230X-10-98] [PMID: 20738844]

[41] Chalasani N, Younossi Z, Lavine JE, *et al.* The diagnosis and management of non-alcoholic fatty liver disease: practice Guideline by the American Association for the Study of Liver Diseases, American College of Gastroenterology, and the American Gastroenterological Association. Hepatology 2012; 55(6): 2005-23.
[http://dx.doi.org/10.1002/hep.25762] [PMID: 22488764]

[42] Fan JG. Epidemiology of alcoholic and nonalcoholic fatty liver disease in China. J Gastroenterol Hepatol 2013; 28 (Suppl. 1): 11-7.
[http://dx.doi.org/10.1111/jgh.12036] [PMID: 23855290]

[43] Kagansky N, Levy S, Keter D, *et al.* Non-alcoholic fatty liver disease common and benign finding in octogenarian patients. Liver Int 2004; 24(6): 588-94.
[http://dx.doi.org/10.1111/j.1478-3231.2004.0969.x] [PMID: 15566509]

[44] Park SH, Jeon WK, Kim SH, *et al.* Prevalence and risk factors of non-alcoholic fatty liver disease among Korean adults. J Gastroenterol Hepatol 2006; 21(1 Pt 1): 138-43.
[http://dx.doi.org/10.1111/j.1440-1746.2005.04086.x] [PMID: 16706825]

[45] Chen CH, Huang MH, Yang JC, *et al.* Prevalence and etiology of elevated serum alanine aminotransferase level in an adult population in Taiwan. J Gastroenterol Hepatol 2007; 22(9): 1482-9.
[http://dx.doi.org/10.1111/j.1440-1746.2006.04615.x] [PMID: 17716352]

[46] Amarapurkar D, Kamani P, Patel N, *et al.* Prevalence of non-alcoholic fatty liver disease: population based study. Ann Hepatol 2007; 6(3): 161-3.
[PMID: 17786142]

[47] Li H, Wang YJ, Tan K, *et al.* Prevalence and risk factors of fatty liver disease in Chengdu, Southwest China. HBPD INT 2009; 8(4): 377-82.
[PMID: 19666406]

[48] Frith J, Day CP, Henderson E, Burt AD, Newton JL. Non-alcoholic fatty liver disease in older people. Gerontology 2009; 55(6): 607-13.
[http://dx.doi.org/10.1159/000235677] [PMID: 19690397]

[49] Caldwell SH, Oelsner DH, Iezzoni JC, Hespenheide EE, Battle EH, Driscoll CJ. Cryptogenic cirrhosis: clinical characterization and risk factors for underlying disease. Hepatology 1999; 29(3): 664-9.
[http://dx.doi.org/10.1002/hep.510290347] [PMID: 10051466]

[50] Hashimoto E, Yatsuji S, Tobari M, *et al.* Hepatocellular carcinoma in patients with nonalcoholic steatohepatitis. J Gastroenterol 2009; 44 (Suppl. 19): 89-95.
[http://dx.doi.org/10.1007/s00535-008-2262-x] [PMID: 19148800]

[51]   Kim HJ, Kim HJ, Lee KE, *et al.* Metabolic significance of nonalcoholic fatty liver disease in nonobese, nondiabetic adults. Arch Intern Med 2004; 164(19): 2169-75.
[http://dx.doi.org/10.1001/archinte.164.19.2169] [PMID: 15505132]

[52]   Sorrentino P, Tarantino G, Conca P, *et al.* Silent non-alcoholic fatty liver disease-a clinical-histological study. J Hepatol 2004; 41(5): 751-7.
[http://dx.doi.org/10.1016/j.jhep.2004.07.010] [PMID: 15519647]

[53]   Weston SR, Leyden W, Murphy R, *et al.* Racial and ethnic distribution of nonalcoholic fatty liver in persons with newly diagnosed chronic liver disease. Hepatology 2005; 41(2): 372-9.
[http://dx.doi.org/10.1002/hep.20554] [PMID: 15723436]

[54]   Arun J, Clements RH, Lazenby AJ, Leeth RR, Abrams GA. The prevalence of nonalcoholic steatohepatitis is greater in morbidly obese men compared to women. Obes Surg 2006; 16(10): 1351-8.
[http://dx.doi.org/10.1381/096089206778663715] [PMID: 17059746]

[55]   Browning JD, Szczepaniak LS, Dobbins R, *et al.* Prevalence of hepatic steatosis in an urban population in the United States: impact of ethnicity. Hepatology 2004; 40(6): 1387-95.
[http://dx.doi.org/10.1002/hep.20466] [PMID: 15565570]

[56]   Kallwitz ER, Kumar M, Aggarwal R, *et al.* Ethnicity and nonalcoholic fatty liver disease in an obesity clinic: the impact of triglycerides. Dig Dis Sci 2008; 53(5): 1358-63.
[http://dx.doi.org/10.1007/s10620-008-0234-x] [PMID: 18347982]

[57]   Wagenknecht LE, Scherzinger AL, Stamm ER, *et al.* Correlates and heritability of nonalcoholic fatty liver disease in a minority cohort. Obesity (Silver Spring) 2009; 17(6): 1240-6.
[PMID: 19584882]

[58]   Fischer GE, Bialek SP, Homan CE, Livingston SE, McMahon BJ. Chronic liver disease among Alaska-Native people, 20032004. Am J Gastroenterol 2009; 104(2): 363-70.
[http://dx.doi.org/10.1038/ajg.2008.57] [PMID: 19174808]

[59]   Fan JG, Saibara T, Chitturi S, Kim BI, Sung JJ, Chutaputti A. What are the risk factors and settings for non-alcoholic fatty liver disease in Asia-Pacific? J Gastroenterol Hepatol 2007; 22(6): 794-800.
[http://dx.doi.org/10.1111/j.1440-1746.2007.04952.x] [PMID: 17498218]

[60]   Hsieh SD, Yoshinaga H, Muto T, Sakurai Y, Kosaka K. Health risks among Japanese men with moderate body mass index. Int J Obes Relat Metab Disord 2000; 24(3): 358-62.
[http://dx.doi.org/10.1038/sj.ijo.0801157] [PMID: 10757631]

[61]   Struben VM, Hespenheide EE, Caldwell SH. Nonalcoholic steatohepatitis and cryptogenic cirrhosis within kindreds. Am J Med 2000; 108(1): 9-13.
[http://dx.doi.org/10.1016/S0002-9343(99)00315-0] [PMID: 11059435]

[62]   Schwimmer JB, Celedon MA, Lavine JE, *et al.* Heritability of nonalcoholic fatty liver disease. Gastroenterology 2009; 136(5): 1585-92.
[http://dx.doi.org/10.1053/j.gastro.2009.01.050] [PMID: 19208353]

[63]   Romeo S, Kozlitina J, Xing C, *et al.* Genetic variation in PNPLA3 confers susceptibility to nonalcoholic fatty liver disease. Nat Genet 2008; 40(12): 1461-5.
[http://dx.doi.org/10.1038/ng.257] [PMID: 18820647]

[64]   Kotronen A, Johansson LE, Johansson LM, *et al.* A common variant in PNPLA3, which encodes adiponutrin, is associated with liver fat content in humans. Diabetologia 2009; 52(6): 1056-60.
[http://dx.doi.org/10.1007/s00125-009-1285-z] [PMID: 19224197]

[65]   Speliotes EK, Yerges-Armstrong LM, Wu J, *et al.* Genome-wide association analysis identifies variants associated with nonalcoholic fatty liver disease that have distinct effects on metabolic traits. PLoS Genet 2011; 7(3): e1001324.
[http://dx.doi.org/10.1371/journal.pgen.1001324] [PMID: 21423719]

[66]   Sookoian S, Pirola CJ. Meta-analysis of the influence of I148M variant of patatin-like phospholipase domain containing 3 gene (PNPLA3) on the susceptibility and histological severity of nonalcoholic fatty liver disease. Hepatology 2011; 53(6): 1883-94.
[http://dx.doi.org/10.1002/hep.24283] [PMID: 21381068]

[67]   Marchesini G, Bugianesi E, Forlani G, *et al.* Nonalcoholic fatty liver, steatohepatitis, and the metabolic syndrome. Hepatology 2003; 37(4): 917-23.
[http://dx.doi.org/10.1053/jhep.2003.50161] [PMID: 12668987]

[68]   Leite NC, Salles GF, Araujo AL, Villela-Nogueira CA, Cardoso CR. Prevalence and associated factors of non-alcoholic fatty liver disease in patients with type-2 diabetes mellitus. Liver Int 2009; 29(1): 113-9.
[http://dx.doi.org/10.1111/j.1478-3231.2008.01718.x] [PMID: 18384521]

[69]   Prashanth M, Ganesh HK, Vima MV, *et al.* Prevalence of nonalcoholic fatty liver disease in patients with type 2 diabetes mellitus. J Assoc Physicians India 2009; 57: 205-10.
[PMID: 19588648]

[70]   Hamaguchi M, Kojima T, Takeda N, *et al.* The metabolic syndrome as a predictor of nonalcoholic fatty liver disease. Ann Intern Med 2005; 143(10): 722-8.
[http://dx.doi.org/10.7326/0003-4819-143-10-200511150-00009] [PMID: 16287793]

[71]   Younossi ZM, Stepanova M, Afendy M, *et al.* Changes in the prevalence of the most common causes of chronic liver diseases in the United States from 1988 to 2008. Clin Gastroenterol Hepatol 2011; 9(6): 524-530.e1.
[http://dx.doi.org/10.1016/j.cgh.2011.03.020] [PMID: 21440669]

[72]   Blachier M, Leleu H, Peck-Radosavljevic M, Valla DC, Roudot-Thoraval F. The burden of liver disease in Europe: a review of available epidemiological data. J Hepatol 2013; 58(3): 593-608.
[http://dx.doi.org/10.1016/j.jhep.2012.12.005] [PMID: 23419824]

[73]   Boza C, Riquelme A, Ibañez L, *et al.* Predictors of nonalcoholic steatohepatitis (NASH) in obese patients undergoing gastric bypass. Obes Surg 2005; 15(8): 1148-53.
[http://dx.doi.org/10.1381/0960892055002347] [PMID: 16197788]

[74]   Spaulding L, Trainer T, Janiec D. Prevalence of non-alcoholic steatohepatitis in morbidly obese subjects undergoing gastric bypass. Obes Surg 2003; 13(3): 347-9.
[http://dx.doi.org/10.1381/096089203765887633] [PMID: 12841891]

[75]   Machado M, Marques-Vidal P, Cortez-Pinto H. Hepatic histology in obese patients undergoing bariatric surgery. J Hepatol 2006; 45(4): 600-6.
[http://dx.doi.org/10.1016/j.jhep.2006.06.013] [PMID: 16899321]

[76]   Bellentani S, Saccoccio G, Masutti F, *et al.* Prevalence of and risk factors for hepatic steatosis in Northern Italy. Ann Intern Med 2000; 132(2): 112-7.
[http://dx.doi.org/10.7326/0003-4819-132-2-200001180-00004] [PMID: 10644271]

[77]   Baranova A, Tran TP, Birerdinc A, Younossi ZM. Systematic review: association of polycystic ovary syndrome with metabolic syndrome and non-alcoholic fatty liver disease. Aliment Pharmacol Ther 2011; 33(7): 801-14.
[http://dx.doi.org/10.1111/j.1365-2036.2011.04579.x] [PMID: 21251033]

[78]   Hossain N, Stepanova M, Afendy A, *et al.* Non-alcoholic steatohepatitis (NASH) in patients with polycystic ovarian syndrome (PCOS). Scand J Gastroenterol 2011; 46(4): 479-84.
[http://dx.doi.org/10.3109/00365521.2010.539251] [PMID: 21114431]

[79]   Sanyal AJ, Contos MJ, Sterling RK, *et al.* Nonalcoholic fatty liver disease in patients with hepatitis C is associated with features of the metabolic syndrome. Am J Gastroenterol 2003; 98(9): 2064-71.
[http://dx.doi.org/10.1111/j.1572-0241.2003.07640.x] [PMID: 14499789]

[80]   Liu CJ, Jeng YM, Chen PJ, *et al.* Influence of metabolic syndrome, viral genotype and antiviral therapy on superimposed fatty liver disease in chronic hepatitis C. Antivir Ther (Lond) 2005; 10(3): 405-15.
[PMID: 15918331]

[81]   Wong VW, Wong GL, Choi PC, *et al.* Disease progression of non-alcoholic fatty liver disease: a prospective study with paired liver biopsies at 3 years. Gut 2010; 59(7): 969-74.
[http://dx.doi.org/10.1136/gut.2009.205088] [PMID: 20581244]

[82]   Argo CK, Caldwell SH. Epidemiology and natural history of non-alcoholic steatohepatitis. Clin Liver Dis 2009; 13(4): 511-31.
[http://dx.doi.org/10.1016/j.cld.2009.07.005] [PMID: 19818302]

[83]   Harrison SA, Torgerson S, Hayashi PH. The natural history of nonalcoholic fatty liver disease: a clinical histopathological study. Am J Gastroenterol 2003; 98(9): 2042-7.
[http://dx.doi.org/10.1111/j.1572-0241.2003.07659.x] [PMID: 14499785]

[84]   Ratziu V, Giral P, Charlotte F, *et al.* Liver fibrosis in overweight patients. Gastroenterology 2000; 118(6): 1117-23.
[http://dx.doi.org/10.1016/S0016-5085(00)70364-7] [PMID: 10833486]

[85]   Sanyal AJ, Banas C, Sargeant C, *et al.* Similarities and differences in outcomes of cirrhosis due to nonalcoholic steatohepatitis and hepatitis C. Hepatology 2006; 43(4): 682-9.
[http://dx.doi.org/10.1002/hep.21103] [PMID: 16502396]

[86]   Caldwell SH, Crespo DM, Kang HS, Al-Osaimi AM. Obesity and hepatocellular carcinoma. Gastroenterology 2004; 127(5) (Suppl. 1): S97-S103.
[http://dx.doi.org/10.1053/j.gastro.2004.09.021] [PMID: 15508109]

[87]   Ekstedt M, Franzén LE, Mathiesen UL, *et al.* Long-term follow-up of patients with NAFLD and elevated liver enzymes. Hepatology 2006; 44(4): 865-73.
[http://dx.doi.org/10.1002/hep.21327] [PMID: 17006923]

[88]   Ong JP, Pitts A, Younossi ZM. Increased overall mortality and liver-related mortality in non-alcoholic fatty liver disease. J Hepatol 2008; 49(4): 608-12.
[http://dx.doi.org/10.1016/j.jhep.2008.06.018] [PMID: 18682312]

[89]   Adams LA, Lymp JF, St Sauver J, *et al.* The natural history of nonalcoholic fatty liver disease: a population-based cohort study. Gastroenterology 2005; 129(1): 113-21.
[http://dx.doi.org/10.1053/j.gastro.2005.04.014] [PMID: 16012941]

[90]   Rafiq N, Bai C, Fang Y, *et al.* Long-term follow-up of patients with nonalcoholic fatty liver. Clin Gastroenterol Hepatol 2009; 7(2): 234-8.
[http://dx.doi.org/10.1016/j.cgh.2008.11.005] [PMID: 19049831]

[91]   Zelber-Sagi S, Lotan R, Shlomai A, *et al.* Predictors for incidence and remission of NAFLD in the general population during a seven-year prospective follow-up. J Hepatol 2012; 56(5): 1145-51.
[http://dx.doi.org/10.1016/j.jhep.2011.12.011] [PMID: 22245895]

[92]   Mottin CC, Moretto M, Padoin AV, *et al.* Histological behavior of hepatic steatosis in morbidly obese patients after weight loss induced by bariatric surgery. Obes Surg 2005; 15(6): 788-93.
[http://dx.doi.org/10.1381/0960892054222830] [PMID: 15978148]

[93]   Kim D, Kim WR, Kim HJ, Therneau TM. Association between noninvasive fibrosis markers and mortality among adults with nonalcoholic fatty liver disease in the United States. Hepatology 2013; 57(4): 1357-65.
[http://dx.doi.org/10.1002/hep.26156] [PMID: 23175136]

[94]   Smedile A, Bugianesi E. Steatosis and hepatocellular carcinoma risk. Eur Rev Med Pharmacol Sci 2005; 9(5): 291-3.
[PMID: 16231592]

[95]   Bugianesi E, Leone N, Vanni E, *et al.* Expanding the natural history of nonalcoholic steatohepatitis: from cryptogenic cirrhosis to hepatocellular carcinoma. Gastroenterology 2002; 123(1): 134-40.
[http://dx.doi.org/10.1053/gast.2002.34168] [PMID: 12105842]

[96]   Takuma Y, Nouso K. Nonalcoholic steatohepatitis-associated hepatocellular carcinoma: our case series and literature review. World J Gastroenterol 2010; 16(12): 1436-41.
[http://dx.doi.org/10.3748/wjg.v16.i12.1436] [PMID: 20333782]

[97]   Targher G, Bertolini L, Rodella S, *et al.* Nonalcoholic fatty liver disease is independently associated with an increased incidence of cardiovascular events in type 2 diabetic patients. Diabetes Care 2007; 30(8): 2119-21.
[http://dx.doi.org/10.2337/dc07-0349] [PMID: 17519430]

[98]   Hamaguchi M, Kojima T, Takeda N, *et al.* Nonalcoholic fatty liver disease is a novel predictor of cardiovascular disease. World J Gastroenterol 2007; 13(10): 1579-84.
[http://dx.doi.org/10.3748/wjg.v13.i10.1579] [PMID: 17461452]

[99]   Schwimmer JB, Deutsch R, Behling C, Lavine JE. Fatty liver as a determinant of atherosclerosis. Hepatology 2005; 42: 610A.

[100] Lee DH, Silventoinen K, Hu G, *et al.* Serum gamma-glutamyltransferase predicts non-fatal myocardial infarction and fatal coronary heart disease among 28,838 middle-aged men and women. Eur Heart J 2006; 27(18): 2170-6.
[http://dx.doi.org/10.1093/eurheartj/ehl086] [PMID: 16772340]

[101] Fraser A, Harris R, Sattar N, Ebrahim S, Smith GD, Lawlor DA. Gamma-glutamyltransferase is associated with incident vascular events independently of alcohol intake: analysis of the British Womens Heart and Health Study and Meta-Analysis. Arterioscler Thromb Vasc Biol 2007; 27(12): 2729-35.
[http://dx.doi.org/10.1161/ATVBAHA.107.152298] [PMID: 17932318]

[102] Yun KE, Shin CY, Yoon YS, Park HS. Elevated alanine aminotransferase levels predict mortality from cardiovascular disease and diabetes in Koreans. Atherosclerosis 2009; 205(2): 533-7.
[http://dx.doi.org/10.1016/j.atherosclerosis.2008.12.012] [PMID: 19159884]

[103] Haring R, Wallaschofski H, Nauck M, Dörr M, Baumeister SE, Völzke H. Ultrasonographic hepatic steatosis increases prediction of mortality risk from elevated serum gamma-glutamyl transpeptidase levels. Hepatology 2009; 50(5): 1403-11.
[http://dx.doi.org/10.1002/hep.23135] [PMID: 19670414]

CHAPTER 2

Clinical Manifestations and Diagnosis of NAFLD

István Tornai*

University of Debrecen, Clinical Center, Department of Medicine, Division of Gastroenterology, Debrecen, Hungary

Abstract: The non-alcoholic fatty liver disease (NAFLD) is a significantly increasing cause of chronic liver disease which is strongly associated with obesity and insulin resistance. Due to this association it is considered as the hepatic manifestation of the metabolic syndrome. According to the emerging clinical and epidemiological data patients with NAFLD have an increased morbidity and mortality of cardiovascular diseases (CVD), type 2 diabetes mellitus, chronic kidney disease as well as malignancies, beyond the liver-related mortality. A number of other less established comorbidities can also manifest together with NAFLD, like colorectal cancer, hypothyroidism, obstructive sleep apnea, polycystic ovarian syndrome and osteoporosis.

The majority of the patients however, maybe asymptomatic and the diagnosis is made only incidentally. Obesity, high body mass index (BMI), elevated transaminase levels and/or hyperechogenic ultrasound form the basis for the diagnosis. About 20% of the cases can progress to non-alcoholic steatohepatitis (NASH) and cirrhosis. Fibrosis, however, can be initiated either in simple steatosis or in NASH *i.e.* due to the most recent results, fibrosis progression is independent of the presence of NASH. In patients with simple steatosis and no inflammation, the fibrosis progression is very slow. The rapid progressors, however, can progress to cirrhosis within 2-6 years. In these patients, hypertension and diabetes are usually also present. The presence and severity of fibrosis on liver biopsy are the best indicators of long-term liver-related outcome in patients with NAFLD. The most important step during diagnosis is risk stratification.

Once a patient with NAFLD develops cirrhosis, he has the same natural history as with other etiologies. Patients with compensated cirrhosis have a 3-4% risk of mortality annually.

Keywords: Cardiovascular diseases, Chronic kidney disease, Colorectal cancer, Hypothyroidism, Non-alcoholic fatty liver disease, Non-alcoholic steatohepatitis, Obstructive sleep apnea, Osteoporosis.

* **Corresponding author István Tornai:** University of Debrecen, Department of Medicine, Debrecen, Nagyerdei krt. 98. 4032; Tel/Fax: 00-36-52-255.172; E-mail: itornai@med.unideb.hu

Tatjana Ábel & Gabriella Lengyel (Eds.)
All rights reserved-© 2017 Bentham Science Publishers

INTRODUCTION

The definition of non-alcoholic fatty liver disease (NAFLD) requires two conditions: the first and most important is to detect steatosis in the liver and the other is the exclusion of other conditions leading to secondary fat accumulation in the liver, such as alcohol consumption, hepatitis C virus infection (especially genotype 3), use of teratogenic medications (tamoxifen, amiodarone *etc.*), parenteral nutrition, hereditary disorders, severe malnutrition, *etc.* (Table **1**). NAFLD encompasses the entire spectrum of fatty liver disease ranging from fatty liver (NAFL) to steatohepatitis (NASH) and cirrhosis. NAFL is described as the presence of hepatic steatosis with no evidence of hepatocellular injury in the form of ballooning of the hepatocytes or no evidence of fibrosis. The risk of progression to cirrhosis is minimal. NASH is defined as the presence of hepatic steatosis, inflammation with hepatocyte injury with or rarely without fibrosis. This can progress to cirrhosis, and later end-stage liver disease, *i.e.* liver failure and/or liver cancer [1].

Table 1. Common causes of secondary hepatic steatosis.

Excessive consumption of alcohol
Chronic hepatitis C (especially genotype 3)
Wilson's disease
Malnutrition
Parenteral nutrition
Medications (amiodarone, methotrexate, steroids, tamoxifen, valproate, *etc.*)
Hereditary lipid abnormalities (abetalipoproteinaemia, lecithin-cholesterol-acyltransferase deficiency)
Acute fatty liver of pregnancy
HELLP syndrome
Reye's syndrome

In the US, as well as in Europe, NAFL has become the most common cause of chronic liver disease. The proportion of NAFLD among chronic liver diseases rose from 47% to 75% in the last 20 years [2]. This is definitively coupled to the increase of obesity, visceral obesity, type 2 diabetes mellitus (T2DM), insulin resistance (IR) and hypertension in the population of the Western societies, together with the ageing of the population. Beyond these parameters of the metabolic syndrome, patients with NAFLD generally display a number of other co-morbidities, as is listed in Table **2**. It is very important to systematically look for these additional conditions. It is believed, that patients with more risk factors have a risk for more advanced NAFLD. A significant percentage of the patients with NAFLD is asymptomatic and the disease is only diagnosed incidentally, especially at the early stages. Due to the co-morbidities, the clinical symptoms are quite variable. There are several extrahepatic disorders, beyond the liver disease, which can cause symptoms, like cardiovascular diseases (CVD), T2DM, chronic kidney disorders (CKD), *etc.*, and some malignant diseases are also detected at a higher rate [3]. It has been shown, that the cardiovascular mortality as well as deaths due to malignancies are both higher in patients with NAFLD, than the liver-related mortality. In patients with NAFLD the cardiovascular mortality is two-times higher than the liver related mortality. In patients with cirrhosis, the cardiovascular disease is the second cause of death. Patients with NAFLD have 9 times more chances of death than patients in the general population. Interestingly, there is no difference between the cardiovascular mortality in patients with NAFL as compared to NASH [4, 5]. NAFLD is strongly associated with obesity and metabolic syndrome, however, a small percentage of the patients also develops NAFLD despite normal body mass index (BMI). The fact, that NASH can be present in lean patients, makes this picture even more complex [6]. The details of the clinical manifestations of NAFLD, except diabetes mellitus, will be discussed in this chapter.

Table 2. Comorbidities associated with NAFLD.

Type 2 diabetes mellitus
Metabolic syndrome
Cardiovascular diseases
Chronic kidney disease
Malignant diseases
Polycystic ovarian syndrome
Chronic obstructive apnea
Hypogonadism
Hypothyroidism
Vitamin D deficiency, osteoporosis

Extrahepatic Complications of NAFLD

Cardiovascular Disorders and NAFLD

Patients affected by NAFLD have a higher risk of developing cardiovascular (CV) events and deaths [7]. One of the most important questions is whether this is only a timely correlation based on underlying risk factors that are present in either conditions, or an independent contribution of NAFLD in the development of

CVD. There are several convincing clinical data on the role of NAFLD in CVD. Both in cross-sectional and follow-up studies, NAFLD has been shown to be an independent risk factor for subclinical coronary heart disease (CHD). It has been reported, that NAFLD is associated with circulatory endothelial dysfunction, independently of classical risk factors for CHD, like obesity, hypertension, diabetes mellitus, *etc.* [8 - 10]. Another sign of early coronary atherosclerosis, like increased coronary artery calcium is also associated with NAFLD, independent of traditional CVD risk factors. This was demonstrated in several studies [11 - 14]. Abnormally reduced coronary flow reserve, another marker of subclinical CHD, was also reported in patients with NAFLD, again independently from conventional CHD risk factors [15]. The presence of reduced coronary flow reserve in patients with NAFLD suggests that decreased coronary flow reserve might represent an additional pathogenic mechanism involved in CHD mortality and morbidity in this group of patients.

Beyond subclinical CHD, accumulating evidence also suggests that there is a strong correlation between NAFLD and clinically manifest CHD. It was reported, that NAFLD was the strongest positive predictor of CHD in patients who had coronary angiography [16]. These data have been confirmed in patients from Europe as well as from Asia [17]. NAFLD proved to be an independent risk factor for CHD, furthermore, there was a significant association with the angiographic severity of CHD [18]. Either biochemically (elevated liver enzymes) or imaging (ultrasound) diagnosed NAFLD, in several prospective studies, was independently associated with an increased risk of fatal or non-fatal CHD events [19 - 21]. Finally, in some studies, including biopsy proven NAFLD cases, during a long follow-up period, a significantly increased CVD mortality as well as liver-related mortality has been observed [5, 22].

Other aspects of CVD have also been investigated, like congestive heart failure or cardiac arrhythmias. In a population-based study of about 3500 men aged between 60 to 79 years have been followed for a mean period of 9 years. Elevated GGT level was associated with significantly increased risk of cardiac failure, even after adjusting for established risk factors for heart failure [23]. Atrial fibrillation is the most common arrhythmia in clinical practice. It has been shown in the Framingham Study, that patients with elevated ALT or AST levels had an increased risk of atrial fibrillation. During a 10-year follow-up period 383 out of 3744 subjects have developed atrial fibrillation [24].

According to the accumulating evidence, NAFLD is involved in the pathophysiology of CHD, through insulin resistance, dyslipidaemia, several pro-inflammatory mediators (like C-reactive protein, interleukin-6, tumor necrosis factor-alpha), or pro-coagulant factors (fibrinogen, factor VIII, plasminogen activator inhibitor [25, 26].

Chronic Kidney Disease and NAFLD

The prevalence of chronic kidney disease (CKD) is gradually increasing year by year in the general population. It is well known that hypertension and diabetes mellitus are the two major independent risk factors for CKD. However, now there is an increasing body of evidence that NAFLD became also a risk factor for CKD [27].

Several large retrospective cross-sectional studies evaluated the relationship between CKD and NAFLD. CKD was defined either by a low glomerular filtration rate (<60 ml/min/1.73 m2) or by proteinuria. The prevalence of CKD in patients with NAFLD was between 21% and 54% while it ranged from 3.7% to 24.2% in patients without NAFLD [28, 29]. In the majority of these studies NAFLD was independently associated with CKD, even after adjusting for age, sex, hypertension, diabetes, BMI, hyperlipidaemia as the most important risk factors for CKD [30, 31]. In these studies, the diagnosis of NAFLD was based on different criteria, either biochemistry, or ultrasonography or rarely biopsy.

There were several prospective studies, evaluating the relation of CKD to NAFLD [32, 33]. In all of these studies the presence of CKD was excluded at baseline, *i.e.* normal GFR and urine analysis. The duration of follow-up ranged between 3-19 years. Four out of these five studies have found NAFLD as an independent risk factor for the development of CKD during the observational period.

Osteoporosis and NAFLD

There is increasing evidence, that NAFLD and osteoporosis are associated to each other. Low bone mineral density (BMD) has been detected in both men and women with metabolic syndrome and NAFLD. Moreover, it seems that an increased risk of osteoporotic fracture is also present in patients with NAFLD. In a recent cross-sectional study from Korea, Moon and coworkers demonstrated that BMD is significantly reduced in postmenopausal women with NAFLD when compared to postmenopausal women without NAFLD. The significance remained after correction of BMI, smoking, age, metabolic syndrome, proving that NAFLD is an independent risk for osteoporosis [34]. Furthermore, it is of concern that similar data have been obtained in obese children and adolescents. Pardee *et al.* demonstrated that obese children with NAFLD have lower BMD, than obese children without fatty liver. In the investigated population 45% of the children had lower than normal BMD, compared to none in the control group [35].

The mechanism of the bone disease in NAFLD is not completely understood. There are several hypotheses. Cytokines released by the inflamed liver might alter bone metabolism, vitamin D deficiency has been demonstrated in NAFLD and the reduced physical activity can have a role, too. Since the decreased BMD can be detected in the early stage of NAFLD, already in children, the role of tumor necrosis factor (TNF) alpha has been raised, since it is elevated in NAFLD and inhibits the activity of the osteoblasts and decreases the osteoclast activity [36]. Furthermore, there are data on bone metabolism, like level of osteoprotegerin, osteopontin *etc.* that are significantly altered in NAFLD [37, 38].

In a recent publication, significantly reduced vitamin D level has been detected. After correction for age, BMI, gender, cardiovascular disease, hypertension, kidney disease, the low level of vitamin D proved to be an independent risk factor for the development of NAFLD [39].

Reduced physical activity, reduced exposure to sunlight and dietary factors together might result in lower level of vitamin D in NAFLD. It has also been demonstrated, that an increased physical activity and weight loss can improve BMD in children [40].

Endocrinopathies

The association of NAFLD and endocrinopathies is based on only retrospective cohort studies and data are limited.

Hypothyroidism

There are several studies where a significantly increased prevalence of hypothyroidism (21 *vs.* 9,5%) was reported in patients with either biopsy or ultrasound proven NAFLD as compared to controls, matched for age, sex and BMI. The association of NAFLD and hypothyroidism was independent of diabetes, age, hypertension and dyslipidaemia, *i.e.* the metabolic risk factors [41].

Polycystic Ovarian Syndrome

Patients with polycystic ovarian syndrome (PCOS) have an increased risk of NAFLD, according to a study [42]. However, in another study in patients with NAFLD a significantly higher prevalence of PCOS was found [43].

Obstructive Sleep Apnea Syndrome

According to a recent review and meta-analysis, there is a significant association between NAFLD and obstructive sleep apnea syndrome (OSAS) [44]. The prevalence of OSAS is 2-4% in Western countries and that is increasing as the body weight increases in the population. OSAS has been associated with obesity, hypertension and insulin resistance, the same metabolic factors which also have a role in the pathogenesis of NAFLD. Repetitive episodes of hypoxia occurring during sleep can contribute to the development of NAFLD. Furthermore, oxygen supply to these patients can reduce the liver enzymes.

Carcinogenesis and NAFLD

One of the largest ever prospective studies of obesity and cancer was published in 2003 [45]. 900.000 US adults were followed for 16 years, from 1982. Mortality of 10 different cancers was found to be significantly elevated in patients with a BMI >35. The risk of cancers ranged mostly between 1.5 and 4.0. The pattern of malignant diseases was somewhat different in females and males. In both men and women, higher BMI was associated with higher mortality due to esophagus, colon and rectum, gallbladder, liver, pancreas, kidney cancer, multiple myeloma and non-Hodgkin's lymphoma. In women, breast, uterine and ovarian cancers were also elevated if BMI was high. In men similar trend for stomach and prostate cancer could be observed. In this study the prevalence of NASH has not been evaluated directly, however, it seems quite obvious, that the possibility of metabolic syndrome as well as NAFLD in that particular population could also be high. The direct investigation of the association of NAFLD and the different cancers, except hepatocellular carcinoma, are limited. Among those only the colorectal cancer has been investigated in several retrospective cross-sectional studies.

Colorectal Cancer

In a Korean study involving 5517 women, a 2-fold increase of adenomatous polyps and 3-fold increase in colorectal cancer in patients with NAFLD were observed as compared to healthy controls [46]. Similarly, in a large European study again an independent association of NAFLD and colorectal adenoma as well as colorectal cancer has been reported [47]. Another retrospective Chinese study investigated patients with NAFLD either with magnetic resonance spectroscopy or histologically. They reported a significantly increased prevalence of colorectal adenomas (34.7% *vs.* 21.5%) as well as colorectal cancer (18.6% *vs.* 5.5%) in patients with NAFLD than in healthy individuals [48]. Furthermore, this association was observed in patients with NASH and no such alteration was seen in patients with simple fatty liver. Even after correction for metabolic and demographic risk factors, NASH patients had a significantly higher risk of both benign and malignant lesions (OR 4.89 and 5.34). Additional observation was that the lesions appeared mostly in the proximal colon and at a younger than expected age. According to this, one can hypothesize the role of liver inflammation and cytokines in carcinogenesis.

Progression of Liver Disease in NAFLD

There is consensus, that the majority of patients with NAFL, *i.e.* simple steatosis usually have a very slow histological progression, however, patients with NASH can progress to cirrhosis. The long-term overall mortality in patients with NAFLD proved to be about 26%, which was about 50% higher as compared to the general population, matched for age and gender. The liver-related mortality was the third cause of death in about 5% of the patients. CVD and malignancies were the two leading causes of death as it has already been mentioned earlier. The long-term liver related prognosis depends mostly on the stage of the liver disease. The more advanced the disease stage at diagnosis, the more patient progresses to end-stage and die due to liver-related causes. Several studies supported the concept, that the presence and severity of fibrosis on liver biopsy would be the most important prognostic factors of long-term survival of patients with NAFLD. In a Swedish study, 118 patients with biopsy-confirmed NAFLD were followed for a median of 21 years [49]. In patients who died, the incidence of advanced fibrosis (>F2) was significantly higher than in survivors (68% *vs.* 28%, P<0.001). Other recent studies have confirmed that liver –related mortality correlated best with the stage of fibrosis [50].

Patients with Risk of Progression

Since patients with NAFLD, especially with NASH can progress to cirrhosis, one of the most important questions is, whether which patient will progress and who will have stable disease. The risk of fibrosis progression has been assessed in several cohort studies and in a meta-analysis [51]. In these studies the patients have not been treated and a repeat liver biopsy was performed after a long follow-up period. It appeared that in patients with NAFLD, the fibrosis progression was generally slow, since it took about 14 years to progress form stage 0 to stage 1 fibrosis. The same progression in patients with NASH happened only in 7 years on average. When stage 0 and 1 patients were investigated together, the annual progression was the same for the patients either with NASH or NAFL. About 20% of the patients however, progressed from stage 0, to stage 3 or 4, within 2-6 years. These rapid progressors need special attention. Again, there was no difference, concerning rapid progressors, between the NAFL or NASH groups. This is very important observation, since it questions the previous concept, that the classical NASH lesions, like ballooning degeneration and lobular inflammation are the major predictors of fibrogenesis. There are several non-histological predictors, like age, BMI, diabetes mellitus type 2, metabolic syndrome. Among the laboratory tests a low platelet count and high and/or raising FIB-4 score are the most important factors to possibly identify the progressors.

Cirrhotic NASH

In most studies about 20% of the patients with NAFLD have bridging fibrosis or cirrhosis. The outcome of patients with cirrhotic NASH has been investigated only in a few studies. The largest study included 152 subjects with cirrhotic NASH and in the control arm patients with hepatitis C virus (HCV) induced cirrhosis were included [52]. In this study patients with compensated cirrhosis had a 3.5-4% annual risk of mortality. Patients with NASH cirrhosis had higher CVD mortality than patients with HCV. Creatinine level proved to be an independent predictor of mortality.

Generally, the first sign of liver failure was the presence of ascites in patients with NASH. It occurred at a slower rate than in subjects with HCV related cirrhosis. Hepatic encephalopathy and variceal hemorrhage however, showed similar rate in both cohorts.

Alcohol and NAFLD

Alcohol consumption is generally considered as having deleterious effect on chronic liver diseases, especially in patients with HCV infection, diabetes mellitus, obesity or metabolic syndrome. However, recently a safe threshold level of alcohol consumption for chronic liver disease has been identified by an Italian study group [53]. It is also known and accepted, that a moderate regular alcohol intake (20-30 g/day) reduces the risk of CVD morbidity and mortality. As we have discussed previously, CVD is the leading cause of mortality in patients with NAFLD, which is two-fold higher than the liver related mortality. Moderate alcohol consumption has been shown to improve metabolic risk factors related to CVD and to protect from NASH and NAFLD [54]. Furthermore, in a recent study there was an inverse correlation between alcohol consumption and carotid artery plaques and stenosis in men with NAFLD. This finding was independent from age, smoking and metabolic syndrome [55]. According to these studies 2-3 drinks per day seem to be safe and perhaps beneficial in patients with NAFLD and NASH.

NASH in Lean Patients

NAFLD is strongly associated with obesity and metabolic syndrome. However, NAFLD can develop in small group of patients with normal body mass index (BMI), too. Most of these patients have been reported from Asia, where visceral obesity, characterized by waist circumference is considered much more important, than BMI. The prevalence of NAFLD has been reported between 7-21% in patients with BMI <25 kg/m^2. The outcome of NAFLD in lean patients is generally good; they less likely progress to cirrhosis [56]. The pathomechanism of NAFLD in lean patients is not well understood. Genetic factors, sudden weight gain, central obesity, *etc.* can play a role in it [57 - 59]. Since it rarely progresses to cirrhosis, biopsy is usually not indicated in these patients.

Diagnosis of NAFLD

The diagnosis of NAFLD requires several important data. Hepatic steatosis should be detected either by imaging or histologically. Furthermore the significant alcohol consumption, other etiology of steatosis as well as other causes of chronic liver disease must be excluded (see Table **1** and **2**). The majority of the patients are either completely asymptomatic or have some specific complaints, like fatigue or abdominal discomfort. Therefore, most of the patients will have a diagnosis incidentally. The aminotransferase levels can be either normal or mildly elevated with some fluctuation. During differential diagnosis chronic viral hepatitis, autoimmune hepatitis, Wilson's disease, haemochromatosis have to be excluded. Mild serum ferritin elevation is frequently seen in patients with NAFLD, sometimes it needs investigation for genetic haemochromatosis. Elevated autoantibodies, like anti-nuclear antibody or smooth muscle antibody, are also seen about 20-30% of the cases and are generally considered as an epiphenomenon.

The most frequent method for diagnosing NAFLD is abdominal ultrasound. It has reasonable specificity and sensitivity. However, mild steatosis sometimes cannot be detected, since ultrasound is reliable for steatosis if the lipid content is higher than 30%, whereas the normal level is below 5%. Magnetic resonance is more accurate, but costly and the availability is also limited. A recent non-invasive and less expensive method, using the transient elastography equipment is the controlled attenuation parameter (CAP) which can accurately measure steatosis and fibrosis together.

Stratification of patients with NAFLD is the most important clinical question, since the majority of patients with NAFLD have a benign course, whereas a small group of patients with NASH, but a minority even without NASH can progress to cirrhosis (rapid progressors). The gold standard is liver biopsy, to evaluate the outcome, but due to the increasing prevalence of NAFLD, non-invasive markers are also developed for the detection of patients with fibrosis. The NAFLD Fibrosis Score is calculated from six parameters, like age, BMI, glucose level, platelet count, AST/ALT ratio and albumin. There are several other non-invasive fibrosis markers, like FIB-4, APRI, and BARD (1).

In those patients, who have a high risk of NASH, liver biopsy is necessary. Patients with a liver stiffness measurement >9.6 kPa, persistently elevated ALT, tender hepatomegaly or with unexplained fatigue are usually also candidate for a histological evaluation.

CONFLICT OF INTEREST

The author confirms that author has no conflict of interest to declare for this publication.

ACKNOWLEDGEMENTS

Declared none.

REFERENCES

[1]   Chalasani N, Younossi Z, Lavine JE, *et al.* The diagnosis and management of non-alcoholic fatty liver disease: practice guideline by the American Gastroenterological Association, American Association for the Study of Liver Diseases, and American College of Gastroenterology. Gastroenterology 2012; 142(7): 1592-609.
      [http://dx.doi.org/10.1053/j.gastro.2012.04.001] [PMID: 22656328]

[2]   Younossi ZM, Stepanova M, Afendy M, *et al.* Changes in the prevalence of the most common causes of chronic liver diseases in the United States from 1988 to 2008. Clin Gastroenterol Hepatol 2011; 9(6): 524-530.e1.
      [http://dx.doi.org/10.1016/j.cgh.2011.03.020] [PMID: 21440669]

[3]   Armstrong MJ, Adams LA, Canbay A, Syn WK. Extrahepatic complications of nonalcoholic fatty liver disease. Hepatology 2014; 59(3): 1174-97.
      [http://dx.doi.org/10.1002/hep.26717] [PMID: 24002776]

[4]   Adams LA, Lymp JF, St Sauver J, *et al.* The natural history of nonalcoholic fatty liver disease: a population-based cohort study. Gastroenterology 2005; 129(1): 113-21.
      [http://dx.doi.org/10.1053/j.gastro.2005.04.014] [PMID: 16012941]

[5]   Rafiq N, Bai C, Fang Y, *et al.* Long-term follow-up of patients with nonalcoholic fatty liver. Clin Gastroenterol Hepatol 2009; 7(2): 234-8.
      [http://dx.doi.org/10.1016/j.cgh.2008.11.005] [PMID: 19049831]

[6]   Wong VW, Chu WC, Wong GL, *et al.* Prevalence of non-alcoholic fatty liver disease and advanced fibrosis in Hong Kong Chinese: a population study using proton-magnetic resonance spectroscopy and transient elastography. Gut 2012; 61(3): 409-15.
[http://dx.doi.org/10.1136/gutjnl-2011-300342] [PMID: 21846782]

[7]   Ballestri S, Lonardo A, Bonapace S, Byrne CD, Loria P, Targher G. Risk of cardiovascular, cardiac and arrhythmic complications in patients with non-alcoholic fatty liver disease. World J Gastroenterol 2014; 20(7): 1724-45.
[http://dx.doi.org/10.3748/wjg.v20.i7.1724] [PMID: 24587651]

[8]   Villanova N, Moscatiello S, Ramilli S, *et al.* Endothelial dysfunction and cardiovascular risk profile in nonalcoholic fatty liver disease. Hepatology 2005; 42(2): 473-80.
[http://dx.doi.org/10.1002/hep.20781] [PMID: 15981216]

[9]   Salvi P, Ruffini R, Agnoletti D, *et al.* Increased arterial stiffness in nonalcoholic fatty liver disease: the Cardio-GOOSE study. J Hypertens 2010; 28(8): 1699-707.
[http://dx.doi.org/10.1097/HJH.0b013e32833a7de6] [PMID: 20467324]

[10]   Pacifico L, Anania C, Martino F, *et al.* Functional and morphological vascular changes in pediatric nonalcoholic fatty liver disease. Hepatology 2010; 52(5): 1643-51.
[http://dx.doi.org/10.1002/hep.23890] [PMID: 20890890]

[11]   Chen CH, Nien CK, Yang CC, Yeh YH. Association between nonalcoholic fatty liver disease and coronary artery calcification. Dig Dis Sci 2010; 55(6): 1752-60.
[http://dx.doi.org/10.1007/s10620-009-0935-9] [PMID: 19688595]

[12]   Jung DH, Lee YJ, Ahn HY, Shim JY, Lee HR. Relationship of hepatic steatosis and alanine aminotransferase with coronary calcification. Clin Chem Lab Med 2010; 48(12): 1829-34.
[http://dx.doi.org/10.1515/CCLM.2010.349] [PMID: 20961204]

[13]   Kim D, Choi SY, Park EH, *et al.* Nonalcoholic fatty liver disease is associated with coronary artery calcification. Hepatology 2012; 56(2): 605-13.
[http://dx.doi.org/10.1002/hep.25593] [PMID: 22271511]

[14]   Sung KC, Wild SH, Kwag HJ, Byrne CD. Fatty liver, insulin resistance, and features of metabolic syndrome: relationships with coronary artery calcium in 10,153 people. Diabetes Care 2012; 35(11): 2359-64.
[http://dx.doi.org/10.2337/dc12-0515] [PMID: 22829522]

[15]   Yilmaz Y, Kurt R, Yonal O, *et al.* Coronary flow reserve is impaired in patients with nonalcoholic fatty liver disease: association with liver fibrosis. Atherosclerosis 2010; 211(1): 182-6.
[http://dx.doi.org/10.1016/j.atherosclerosis.2010.01.049] [PMID: 20181335]

[16]   Mirbagheri SA, Rashidi A, Abdi S, Saedi D, Abouzari M. Liver: an alarm for the heart? Liver Int 2007; 27(7): 891-4.
[http://dx.doi.org/10.1111/j.1478-3231.2007.01531.x] [PMID: 17696926]

[17]   Wong VW, Wong GL, Yip GW, *et al.* Coronary artery disease and cardiovascular outcomes in patients with non-alcoholic fatty liver disease. Gut 2011; 60(12): 1721-7.
[http://dx.doi.org/10.1136/gut.2011.242016] [PMID: 21602530]

[18]   Domanski JP, Park SJ, Harrison SA. Cardiovascular disease and nonalcoholic fatty liver disease: does histologic severity matter? J Clin Gastroenterol 2012; 46(5): 427-30.
[http://dx.doi.org/10.1097/MCG.0b013e31822fb3f7] [PMID: 22469639]

[19]   Goessling W, Massaro JM, Vasan RS, DAgostino RB Sr, Ellison RC, Fox CS. Aminotransferase levels and 20-year risk of metabolic syndrome, diabetes, and cardiovascular disease. Gastroenterology 2008; 135(6): 1935-1944, 1944.e1.
[http://dx.doi.org/10.1053/j.gastro.2008.09.018] [PMID: 19010326]

[20]   Dunn W, Xu R, Wingard DL, *et al.* Suspected nonalcoholic fatty liver disease and mortality risk in a population-based cohort study. Am J Gastroenterol 2008; 103(9): 2263-71.
[http://dx.doi.org/10.1111/j.1572-0241.2008.02034.x] [PMID: 18684196]

[21]   Targher G, Bertolini L, Rodella S, *et al.* Nonalcoholic fatty liver disease is independently associated with an increased incidence of cardiovascular events in type 2 diabetic patients. Diabetes Care 2007; 30(8): 2119-21.
[http://dx.doi.org/10.2337/dc07-0349] [PMID: 17519430]

[22]   Ekstedt M, Franzén LE, Mathiesen UL, *et al.* Long-term follow-up of patients with NAFLD and elevated liver enzymes. Hepatology 2006; 44(4): 865-73.
[http://dx.doi.org/10.1002/hep.21327] [PMID: 17006923]

[23]   Wannamethee SG, Whincup PH, Shaper AG, Lennon L, Sattar N. Γ-glutamyltransferase, hepatic enzymes, and risk of incident heart failure in older men. Arterioscler Thromb Vasc Biol 2012; 32(3): 830-5.
[http://dx.doi.org/10.1161/ATVBAHA.111.240457] [PMID: 22223732]

[24]   Sinner MF, Wang N, Fox CS, *et al.* Relation of circulating liver transaminase concentrations to risk of new-onset atrial fibrillation. Am J Cardiol 2013; 111(2): 219-24.
[http://dx.doi.org/10.1016/j.amjcard.2012.09.021] [PMID: 23127690]

[25]   Papatheodoridis GV, Chrysanthos N, Cholongitas E, *et al.* Thrombotic risk factors and liver histologic lesions in non-alcoholic fatty liver disease. J Hepatol 2009; 51(5): 931-8.
[http://dx.doi.org/10.1016/j.jhep.2009.06.023] [PMID: 19726097]

[26]   Targher G, Byrne CD. Diagnosis and management of nonalcoholic fatty liver disease and its hemostatic/thrombotic and vascular complications. Semin Thromb Hemost 2013; 39(2): 214-28.
[http://dx.doi.org/10.1055/s-0033-1334866] [PMID: 23397556]

[27]   Musso G, Gambino R, Tabibian JH. Association of non-alcoholic fatty liver disease with chronic kidney disease: a systematic review and meta-analysis. PLoS Med 2014; 11(7): e1001680.
[http://dx.doi.org/10.1371/journal.pmed.1001680]

[28]   Targher G, Pichiri I, Zoppini G, Trombetta M, Bonora E. Increased prevalence of chronic kidney disease in patients with Type 1 diabetes and non-alcoholic fatty liver. Diabet Med 2012; 29(2): 220-6.
[http://dx.doi.org/10.1111/j.1464-5491.2011.03427.x] [PMID: 21883436]

[29]   Sirota JC, McFann K, Targher G, Chonchol M, Jalal DI. Association between nonalcoholic liver disease and chronic kidney disease: an ultrasound analysis from NHANES 19881994. Am J Nephrol 2012; 36(5): 466-71.
[http://dx.doi.org/10.1159/000343885] [PMID: 23128368]

[30]   Targher G, Bertolini L, Chonchol M, *et al.* Non-alcoholic fatty liver disease is independently associated with an increased prevalence of chronic kidney disease and retinopathy in type 1 diabetic patients. Diabetologia 2010; 53(7): 1341-8.
[http://dx.doi.org/10.1007/s00125-010-1720-1] [PMID: 20369224]

[31]   Hwang ST, Cho YK, Yun JW, *et al.* Impact of non-alcoholic fatty liver disease on microalbuminuria in patients with prediabetes and diabetes. Intern Med J 2010; 40(6): 437-42.
[http://dx.doi.org/10.1111/j.1445-5994.2009.01979.x] [PMID: 19460054]

[32]   Ryu S, Chang Y, Kim DI, Kim WS, Suh BS. gamma-Glutamyltransferase as a predictor of chronic kidney disease in nonhypertensive and nondiabetic Korean men. Clin Chem 2007; 53(1): 71-7.
[http://dx.doi.org/10.1373/clinchem.2006.078980] [PMID: 17110470]

[33]   Targher G, Chonchol M, Bertolini L, *et al.* Increased risk of CKD among type 2 diabetics with nonalcoholic fatty liver disease. J Am Soc Nephrol 2008; 19(8): 1564-70.
[http://dx.doi.org/10.1681/ASN.2007101155] [PMID: 18385424]

[34]   Moon S-S, Lee Y-S, Kim SW. Association of nonalcoholic fatty liver disease with low bone mass in postmenopausal women. Endocrine 2012; 42(2): 423-9.
[http://dx.doi.org/10.1007/s12020-012-9639-6] [PMID: 22407492]

[35]   Pardee PE, Dunn W, Schwimmer JB. Non-alcoholic fatty liver disease is associated with low bone mineral density in obese children. Aliment Pharmacol Ther 2012; 35(2): 248-54.
[http://dx.doi.org/10.1111/j.1365-2036.2011.04924.x] [PMID: 22111971]

[36]   Lima-Cabello E, García-Mediavilla MV, Miquilena-Colina ME, *et al.* Enhanced expression of pro-inflammatory mediators and liver X-receptor-regulated lipogenic genes in non-alcoholic fatty liver disease and hepatitis C. Clin Sci 2011; 120(6): 239-50.
[http://dx.doi.org/10.1042/CS20100387] [PMID: 20929443]

[37]   Yilmaz Y. Review article: non-alcoholic fatty liver disease and osteoporosis clinical and molecular crosstalk. Aliment Pharmacol Ther 2012; 36(4): 345-52.
[http://dx.doi.org/10.1111/j.1365-2036.2012.05196.x] [PMID: 22730920]

[38]   Yilmaz Y, Yonal O, Kurt R, *et al.* Serum levels of osteoprotegerin in the spectrum of nonalcoholic fatty liver disease. Scand J Clin Lab Invest 2010; 70(8): 541-6.
[http://dx.doi.org/10.3109/00365513.2010.524933] [PMID: 20942739]

[39]   Jablonski KL, Jovanovich A, Holmen J, *et al.* Low 25-hydroxyvitamin D level is independently associated with non-alcoholic fatty liver disease. Nutr Metab Cardiovasc Dis 2013; 23(8): 792-8.
[http://dx.doi.org/10.1016/j.numecd.2012.12.006] [PMID: 23415456]

[40]   Campos RM, de Piano A, da Silva PL, *et al.* The role of pro/anti-inflammatory adipokines on bone metabolism in NAFLD obese adolescents: effects of long-term interdisciplinary therapy. Endocrine 2012; 42(1): 146-56.
[http://dx.doi.org/10.1007/s12020-012-9613-3] [PMID: 22315014]

[41]   Pagadala MR, Zein CO, Dasarathy S, Yerian LM, Lopez R, McCullough AJ. Prevalence of hypothyroidism in nonalcoholic fatty liver disease. Dig Dis Sci 2012; 57(2): 528-34.
[http://dx.doi.org/10.1007/s10620-011-2006-2] [PMID: 22183820]

[42]   Zueff LF, Martins WP, Vieira CS, Ferriani RA. Ultrasonographic and laboratory markers of metabolic and cardiovascular disease risk in obese women with polycystic ovary syndrome. Ultrasound Obstet Gynecol 2012; 39(3): 341-7.
[http://dx.doi.org/10.1002/uog.10084] [PMID: 21898634]

[43]   Brzozowska MM, Ostapowicz G, Weltman MD. An association between non-alcoholic fatty liver disease and polycystic ovarian syndrome. J Gastroenterol Hepatol 2009; 24(2): 243-7.
[http://dx.doi.org/10.1111/j.1440-1746.2008.05740.x] [PMID: 19215335]

[44]   Musso G, Cassader M, Olivetti C, Rosina F, Carbone G, Gambino R. Association of obstructive sleep apnoea with the presence and severity of non-alcoholic fatty liver disease. A systematic review and meta-analysis. Obes Rev 2013; 14(5): 417-31.
[http://dx.doi.org/10.1111/obr.12020] [PMID: 23387384]

[45]   Calle EE, Rodriguez C, Walker-Thurmond K, Thun MJ. Overweight, obesity, and mortality from cancer in a prospectively studied cohort of U.S. adults. N Engl J Med 2003; 348(17): 1625-38.
[http://dx.doi.org/10.1056/NEJMoa021423] [PMID: 12711737]

[46]   Lee YI, Lim YS, Park HS. Colorectal neoplasms in relation to non-alcoholic fatty liver disease in Korean women: a retrospective cohort study. J Gastroenterol Hepatol 2012; 27(1): 91-5.
[http://dx.doi.org/10.1111/j.1440-1746.2011.06816.x] [PMID: 21679251]

[47]   Stadlmayr A, Aigner E, Steger B, *et al.* Nonalcoholic fatty liver disease: an independent risk factor for colorectal neoplasia. J Intern Med 2011; 270(1): 41-9.
[http://dx.doi.org/10.1111/j.1365-2796.2011.02377.x] [PMID: 21414047]

[48]   Wong VW, Wong GL, Tsang SW, *et al.* High prevalence of colorectal neoplasm in patients with non-alcoholic steatohepatitis. Gut 2011; 60(6): 829-36.
[http://dx.doi.org/10.1136/gut.2011.237974] [PMID: 21339204]

[49]   Söderberg C, Stål P, Askling J, *et al.* Decreased survival of subjects with elevated liver function tests during a 28-year follow-up. Hepatology 2010; 51(2): 595-602.
[http://dx.doi.org/10.1002/hep.23314] [PMID: 20014114]

[50]   Younossi ZM, Stepanova M, Rafiq N, *et al.* Pathologic criteria for nonalcoholic steatohepatitis: interprotocol agreement and ability to predict liver-related mortality. Hepatology 2011; 53(6): 1874-82.
[http://dx.doi.org/10.1002/hep.24268] [PMID: 21360720]

[51]   Singh S, Allen AM, Wang Z, Prokop LJ, Murad MH, Loomba R. Fibrosis progression in nonalcoholic fatty liver *vs* nonalcoholic steatohepatitis: a systematic review and meta-analysis of paired-biopsy studies. Clin Gastroenterol Hepatol 2015; 13(4): 643-54.e1.
[http://dx.doi.org/10.1016/j.cgh.2014.04.014] [PMID: 24768810]

[52]   Sanyal AJ, Banas C, Sargeant C, *et al.* Similarities and differences in outcomes of cirrhosis due to nonalcoholic steatohepatitis and hepatitis C. Hepatology 2006; 43(4): 682-9.
[http://dx.doi.org/10.1002/hep.21103] [PMID: 16502396]

[53]   Bellentani S, Saccoccio G, Costa G, *et al.* Drinking habits as cofactors of risk for alcohol induced liver damage. Gut 1997; 41(6): 845-50.
[http://dx.doi.org/10.1136/gut.41.6.845] [PMID: 9462221]

[54]   Moriya A, Iwasaki Y, Ohguchi S, *et al.* Roles of alcohol consumption in fatty liver: a longitudinal study. J Hepatol 2015; 62(4): 921-7.
[http://dx.doi.org/10.1016/j.jhep.2014.11.025] [PMID: 25433160]

[55]   Sinn DH, Gwak GY, Cho J, *et al.* Modest alcohol consumption and carotid plaques or carotid artery stenosis in men with non-alcoholic fatty liver disease. Atherosclerosis 2014; 234(2): 270-5.
[http://dx.doi.org/10.1016/j.atherosclerosis.2014.03.001] [PMID: 24704629]

[56]   Wong VW, Vergniol J, Wong GL, *et al.* Diagnosis of fibrosis and cirrhosis using liver stiffness measurement in nonalcoholic fatty liver disease. Hepatology 2010; 51(2): 454-62.
[http://dx.doi.org/10.1002/hep.23312] [PMID: 20101745]

[57]   Petersen KF, Dufour S, Hariri A, *et al.* Apolipoprotein C3 gene variants in nonalcoholic fatty liver disease. N Engl J Med 2010; 362(12): 1082-9.
[http://dx.doi.org/10.1056/NEJMoa0907295] [PMID: 20335584]

[58]   Kechagias S, Ernersson A, Dahlqvist O, Lundberg P, Lindström T, Nystrom FH. Fast-food-based hyper-alimentation can induce rapid and profound elevation of serum alanine aminotransferase in healthy subjects. Gut 2008; 57(5): 649-54.
[http://dx.doi.org/10.1136/gut.2007.131797] [PMID: 18276725]

[59]   Wong VW, Wong GL, Yeung DK, *et al.* Incidence of non-alcoholic fatty liver disease in Hong Kong: a population study with paired proton-magnetic resonance spectroscopy. J Hepatol 2015; 62(1): 182-9.
[http://dx.doi.org/10.1016/j.jhep.2014.08.041] [PMID: 25195550]

CHAPTER 3

Imaging of NAFLD

Zoltán Harmat[*] and Omar Giyab

University of Pécs, Medical School, Department of Radiology, Pécs, Hungary

Abstract: With the epidemic of obesity and metabolic syndrome, NAFLD is affecting a large number of the general population than ever before. Its diagnosis and monitoring can be challenging as it is more common in obese patients. It is a reversible condition, and reaching an early diagnosis could help in preventing and reversing the process. If left untreated, it can advance to liver cirrhosis, and lead to hepatocellular carcinoma in some cases. Therefore, its non-invasive accurate and early diagnosis has a significant importance in both patients and clinicians. Radiology has to offer a wide repertoire of methods that can diagnose and monitor this condition. Biopsy is very accurate, and is the only widely accepted method to distinguish NAFLD from other forms of liver disease, but its inconvenience to the patient and the general risks of invasive procedures limits its clinical use. In addition, biopsy cannot be representative to structural changes in the entire organ. Medical imaging until recent advances was not able to compete with biopsy. Non-invasive diagnostic tests that are used include ultrasonography (sonoelastography), computed tomography, and magnetic resonance imaging. Special MRI sequences (Chemical Shift Imaging, Fast SE Imaging, elastography, spectroscopy), which are capable of providing comparable results to biopsy. In contrast to biopsies, these methods provide a non-invasive way of giving a representative assessment of the whole liver.

Keywords: Cirrhosis, Fat suppression, Fibroscan, Hepatocellular carcinoma, Liver biopsy, Liver CT liver imaging, Liver MRI, Liver ultrasound, MR elastography, MR spectroscopy, Sonoelastography, Steatohepatitis, Steatosis, Steatosis imaging.

INTRODUCTION

Non-alcoholic fatty liver disease (NAFLD) is nowadays the most common cause of abnormality in liver function. Its prevalence in the average population is 9-32%. During the course of the disease there is a significant focal or diffuse accumulation of triglycerides in the hepatocytes.

[*] **Corresponding author Zoltán Harmat:** University of Pécs, Medical School, Department of Radiology, Pécs, Hungary; Tel: +3672535801 E-mail: harmatzoltan@gmail.com

Tatjana Ábel & Gabriella Lengyel (Eds.)
All rights reserved-© 2017 Bentham Science Publishers

Diffuse deposition of fat can be mild, or can progress to steatohepatitis, liver cirrhosis and eventually can lead to hepatocellular carcinoma.

Nowadays, NAFLD is increasingly seen in younger ages, therefore fast, accurate, and non-invasive diagnostic methods are coming to the forefront. This is important for both early diagnosis, and also in the follow-up of treatment response as well.

Biopsy is the most accurate method and is still considered to be the gold standard in determining the extent of fatty infiltration. However, its disadvantages include complications in a small number of cases (<3%). It cannot be representative of structural changes in the liver, and it cannot be repeated indefinitely. At the same time, diagnostic imaging has become more reliable to accurately detect steatosis and determine its stage without the need for any invasive procedure. The diagnostic imaging modalities available for the diagnosis of NAFLD are ultrasound (US), sonoelastography, computed tomography (CT), magnetic resonance imaging (MRI) [1].

IMAGING MODALITIES

Ultrasound

Ultrasound is the most readily available, inexpensive imaging modality, with no ionising radiation involved. A convex transducer with a frequency range of 2-8 MHz is used to examine the liver, but the frequency used is highly dependent on the patient's physique.

The assessment of the liver's echogenicity and the degree of steatosis is very subjective, and operator dependent. Ultrasound is operator dependant, and there can be large variations between examinations performed on different machines, and even a single sonographer is not always able to reproduce previous parameters. The normal liver is homogeneous, has a characteristic echotexture, the echogenicity of which equals to, or is slightly more than that of the kidney and spleen. The liver appears to be homogeneous if examined with a good quality ultrasound, the intrahepatic vessels can be sharply delineated, and the diaphragmatic surface of the liver has a well distinguishable boundary. In fatty infiltration of the liver there is an increased reflection of ultrasound waves, this will result in a "bright liver". In severe fatty infiltration due to the pronounced attenuation of sound waves, the liver structure will become increasingly difficult to assess. The degree of fatty infiltration has three grades on US.

Initially, the fatty deposition increases the echogenicity of the liver (Grade I.), then the contour of the vessels will become blurred (Grade III.), in more severe steatosis the contour of the diaphragmatic surface will become obscured or even masked (Grade III.) (Fig. **1**).

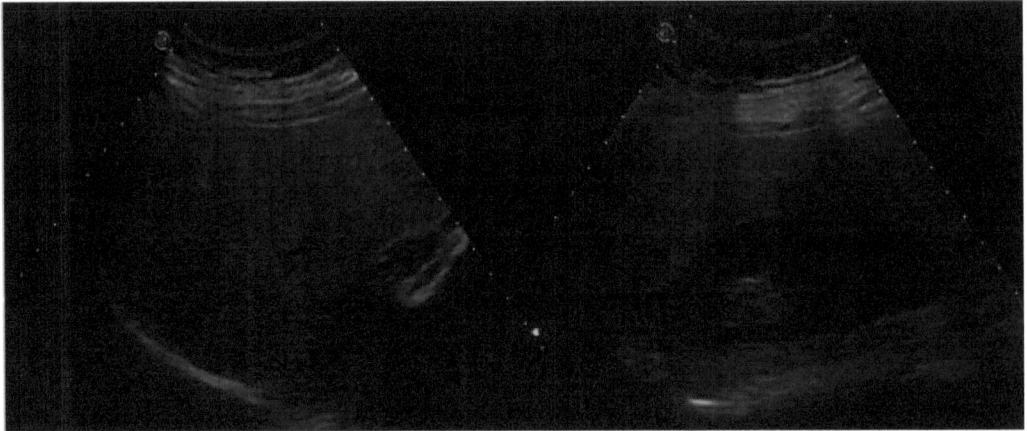

Fig. (1). On ultrasound image severe fatty infiltration of the liver cause pronounced attenuation of sound waves. The echogenicity of the liver is more higher than that of the kidney.

The sensitivity of US with respect to hepatic steatosis is between 60-94%, specificity 84-95% [2]. In the case of marked obesity both the sensitivity (49%) and specificity (75%) decrease. The sensitivity of US is almost 100% when steatosis the liver exceeds 30%, in these cases the differentiation between steatosis and fibrosis is extremely difficult [3].

Sonoelastography

The latest US techniques allow for the assessment of the livers' elasticity. This function is either built into modern US machines (sonoelastography), or a purpose built fibroscan machine can quantitatively determine the stiffness of liver parenchyma.

It is a generally known fact that diseased tissue has different elasticity compared to healthy tissue. This can partly be explained by the amount of extracellular fluid, since after dehydration almost all human tissue will become incompressible.

We can assess tissue elasticity by elastography, which has two different types; strain, and shearwave elastography. Both techniques can be used in several ways. The formers' most common method of implementation is the acoustic radiation force impulse imaging (ARFI), and the latter's is the transient elastography. In ARFI, a high energy focused ultrasound impulse wave is applied; this in turn will cause tissue movement which can then be detected. This method can be most simply applied if the same transducer used to generate the high energy radiofrequency impulse for tissue movement, is also used to generate the lower energy radiofrequency impulse for imaging. The advantage of this technique is that the elasticity of small changes in tissue and focal lesions can be easily evaluated, but larger areas are more difficult to assess. This method is already available in modern US machines; it can be used to assess focal lesions of the liver, breast, and thyroid gland. Transient elastography measures the change in velocity of shear waves; by applying brief vibrational excitations into the tissue. Thus, this method is primarily suitable for determining the average elasticity of larger volumes of tissues, and not for detecting smaller lesions. This technique is also used by the Fibroscan machine, which was specifically developed for the assessment of liver elasticity. Its advantage is that it can rapidly provide accurate information regarding the liver parenchyma, in just 3-5 minutes. For an accurate measurement at least a 6 cm thick liver tissue is needed. Unfortunately, this technique cannot be used if the thickness of the abdominal wall exceeds 2 cm. Both strain, and shearwave elastography provide quantitative results about the current condition of the liver parenchyma. While biopsy which is considered to be the gold standard provides information about only $1/50000^{th}$ of the liver volume, elastography allows for the assessment of about $1/100^{th}$ of the liver volume. Elastography is non-invasive, can be repeated, and allow for the follow up on disease progression. The effectiveness of therapy can be also evaluated in an accurate, quantitative way [4].

The elasticity of normal liver parenchyma is < 6 kPa, and the shear wave velocity is ~ 1 m/s. In steatosis, and moderate fibrosis these values change to 6-12 kPa / 1.7 m/s, in cirrhosis >12.5 kPa, or even 40-70 kPa /3.6-5.0 m/s.

Computed Tomography

Axial plane imaging has an outstanding significance in the diagnostics of both diffuse and focal liver diseases. Multidetector-row, and especially dual energy CT scanners provide excellent morphological images of the liver. It is primarily good for the assessment of focal liver lesions and the anatomy of the liver and surrounding organs. Thanks to the numerous adjustable parameters of the multidetector-row systems, and to the dual energy application, focal and diffuse diseases can be detected well. In these diseases – thanks to the relative affordability of CT exams – it is often the imaging modality of choice.

With the advances in CT, and the emergence of 128-256-320 slice scanners, the lesions can be detected and accurately characterised at earlier stages than ever before. The extent of fatty deposition in the liver can be well determined on a native CT scan, but it is not suitable for the early detection of inflammation, necrosis, or fibrosis. If the extent of fatty deposition in hepatocytes is greater than 30%, the sensitivity of CT is 82%, and the specificity is 100%. The normal density of liver parenchyma is 50 – 75 HU, which is approximately 8 – 10 HU more than that of the spleen. In fatty infiltration, with every milligram of triglyceride deposition, there is a 1.6 HU decrease in the livers' density, and compared to the density of the spleen, the difference will be increasingly bigger [5]. The diagnosis of steatosis can be set if the density of the liver is 10 HU less than that of the spleen, or if the density of the liver is lower than 40 HU (Fig. **2**). The CT scan objectively assesses the extent of hepatic steatosis, the exam is easily reproducible, and thanks to the low dose techniques, its radiation burden is also minimal. The dual energy CT technique is also suitable to set the diagnosis of NAFLD. By examining the liver with a tube voltage of 80 kV and 140 kV, it is possible to calculate the exact degree of steatosis. The absorption of soft X-ray beams by a steatotic liver parenchyma is decreased, while the absorption of hard X-ray beam is increased. When the density difference of the liver parenchyma using a tube voltage of 80 kV and 140 kV is more than 10 HU, then the degree of steatosis is more than 25%.

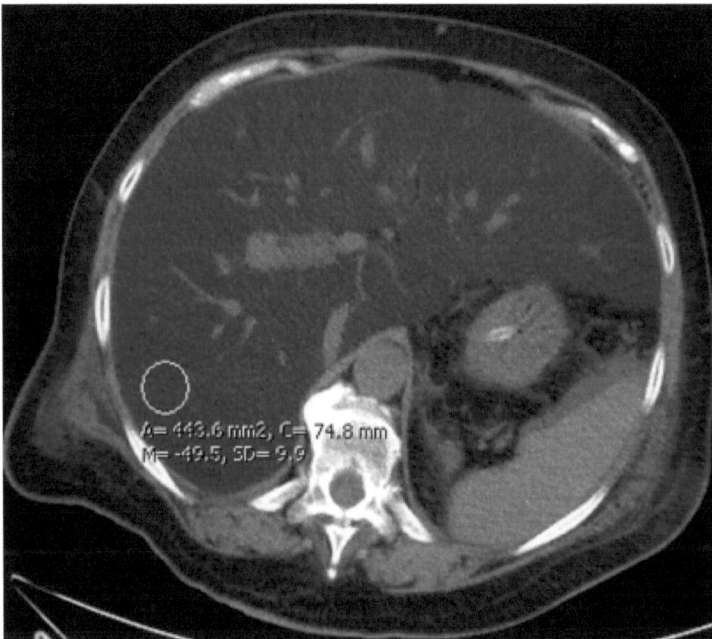

Fig. (2). The native CT image with the very low density (-49,5 HU) of the liver parenchyma can demonstrate high fatty infiltration of the liver.

Contrast enhanced CT is not suitable for the determination of liver fat content. In such cases the changes in the liver and spleen density depends to a great extent on the technique and timing of the acquisition. There is a large overlap between the density values of normal and steatotic liver parenchyma on contrast enhanced CT, therefore an accurate diagnosis cannot be based on this. Xenon CT known for its use in determining cerebral blood flow is showing promising results in the early diagnosis of steatosis. After the inhalation of 25% Xe gas for 4-4 minutes (wash in – wash out) CT scan of the liver is performed every minute to determine the hepatic blood flow. According to the trials, the Xe CT scan sensitively demonstrate changes in hepatic blood flow even at early phases, which correlates well with the degree of steatosis [6].

Magnetic Resonance Imaging

Although MRI of the liver is the most time consuming and expansive modality, yet it is the most accurate in detecting even slight fatty deposition in the liver parenchyma.

On conventional T1-weighted images, increased hepatic fat will result in increased signal intensity, but this has little sensitivity and specificity (Fig. **3**). To determine the fat accumulation inside the liver it is necessary to use special sequences such as chemical shift imaging (CSI), proton spectroscopy, and MR elastography. These techniques are higher than 90% sensitivity and specificity [7].

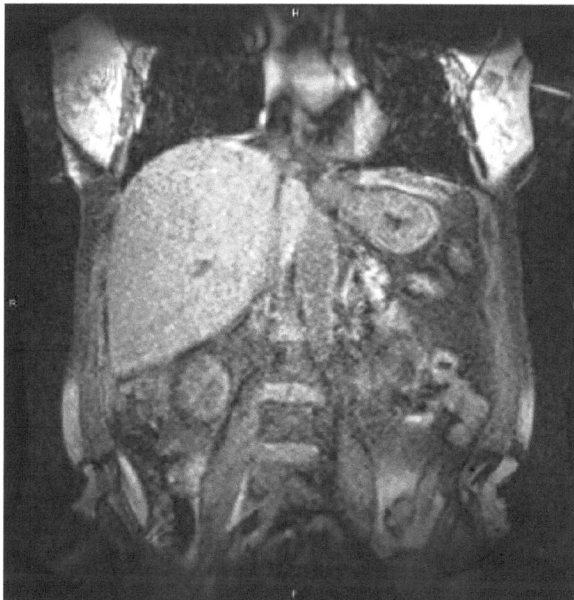

Fig. (3). Conventional T1-weighted images, increased hepatic fat will result in increased signal intensity.

Chemical Shift Imaging

In this sequence fatty infiltration of the liver is accurately quantified by measuring the precession frequency differences between fat ($-CH_2$) and water ($-OH$) protons. When the proton magnetizations are opposed (become out of phase) the difference in frequency results in tissues containing fat and water to lose their signal intensity. In-phase and out-of-phase data are compared and a decreased signal can be seen. These data are obtained from the magnetisation of protons from both water and fat being in-phase to provide a stronger signal. The healthy liver parenchyma shows similar signal on in-phase and out of phase images, but a steatotic liver shows decreased signal intensity on the out-of-phase images. This decrease is more pronounced in steatosis. Breath-hold gradient-echo (GRE) imaging is routinely used to evaluate steatosis, by using tissues like surrounding muscles or even the spleen as a reference. Dixon in 1984 was the pioneer who used a fat-saturated MRI sequence in chemical shift imaging for fat quantification in organs. When compared to out-of phase GRE imaging, fast SE sequences are better for the quantification of hepatic fat, this is especially true in the case of cirrhosis, because GRE sequences are more susceptible to paramagnetic effects of iron in the cirrhotic liver.

Dixon has introduced the two point method for CSI with spin echo (SE) sequence, equalising the rephrasing pulse in SE sequence generate out-of-phase images, while the unamended SE sequence images were considered as in-phase images.

Images show that water and fat are extracted from the subtraction of image sets, and this allows for fat quantification. A so called three point technique received its name after the acquisition of a third image, along with the in-phase and out-of-phase images. This technique has certain limitations such as long acquisition time and sensitivity to the inhomogeneities of the magnetic field. The problem of misregistration and susceptibility to magnetic field inhomogeneities has been addressed by the application of modified dual-echo chemical shift GRE sequences. However, the problem of magnetic field inhomogeneities is not observed with modern scanners utilising shorter echo times (TE), and minimizing the effect of T2* relaxivity. Chemical shift GRE imaging is widely used for assessing steatotic livers. The methods introduced by Dixon allow for the detection of fat content of at least 15% or higher. CSI can assess the whole liver at once. The advantages of the Dixon method include its ability to evaluate the whole liver, its technical simplicity, not involving ionising radiation, and its minimal vulnerability to the interfering factors. The drawbacks of MR fat quantification are the variability of results which differ with different MR systems, and depend on the scanning parameters and the method of analysis. Nevertheless MRI is still expansive, and this limits its use in the follow up on therapy. MR is highly sensitive in the detection of fat, but it is not suitable to determine the absolute fat content of the liver.

Fast SE Imaging

This technique calculates the percentage of hepatic fat from the decrease in the signal intensity of T2-weighted fat-saturated fast SE images, compared to the normal T2-weighted images. The cirrhotic liver parenchyma has an increased iron content compared to the healthy parenchyma, and due to the paramagnetic effect of iron, this will result in magnetic field inhomogeneities and will interfere with the $T2^*$ relaxation. GRE sequences might not be reliable for quantifying fat in the cirrhotic parenchyma. Using T2-weighted fat-saturated and non-fat-saturated fast SE sequences can avoid signal loss that results from $T2^*$ effect. With the newer 3 T magnets, there has been an increase in the usage of MRI for evaluation of liver fat content. The difference in chemical shift between water and fat in a 3 T magnetic field is around 415 Hz, compared to 208 Hz at 1.5 T. Utilising this difference in frequency, TEs at in-phase and out-of-phase GRE imaging with a 3 T magnet are almost half of those that are needed to generate an echo in a 1.5 T magnet.

MR Spectroscopy

The most accurate, non-invasive method for the assessment of fat deposition in the liver is Proton MR spectroscopy (MRS). This method is based on the differences between the T1 and T2 relaxation times of fat and water protons inside the hepatocytes. It requires at least a 3 T system to perform. Direct measurement of lipid resonance peak allows for the quantitative assessment and mapping of fatty infiltration. Unlike many other sequences, MRS is not affected by fibrosis, glycogen, or iron overload. On the other hand it is a complex technique that needs good patient cooperation, and only a small part of the liver can be sampled at one time [8].

MR Elastography

Hepatic fibrosis is strongly correlated to increased stiffness of the liver parenchyma. In fibrosis there is elevated portal venous pressure due to the increased intrahepatic vascular resistance. Originally developed for ultra-sonography, in which elastography is based on compressional radiofrequency impulses. These impulses are made visible with Doppler technique as shear-wave transients propagating through the liver parenchyma, the speed of propagation depending on the elasticity of the parenchyma. MR elastography on the other hand allows for the quantification (not possible with US) of the viscoelastic properties of the liver, this is especially useful for the assessment of hepatic fibrosis. External and sinusoidal vibrational patterns are applied to the liver parenchyma using a 2D GE MR elastography sequence, which uses motion encoding gradients along the section selection direction in order to detect cyclic motion in the through plane direction; the external acoustic driver and motion-encoding gradients needs to be synchronized in both frequency and phase [9].

CONCLUSION

NAFLD is considered to be the hepatic manifestation of the metabolic syndrome, and is the main cause of chronic liver disease and sometimes malfunction. With the increase seen in obesity rates and type 2 diabetes mellitus, NAFLD is expected to rise. Hence, there is an increasing need for techniques that can help in the non- invasive, early diagnosis, and also follow up of NAFLD. Finding a way to accurately produce reproducible results in the estimation of hepatic fat is of utmost importance. Steatosis mostly affects the liver diffusely and homogeneously. Less commonly the liver can be affected in an inhomogeneous fashion with focal deposition of fat in the perivascular or subcapsular areas. Areas of focal sparing are not an infrequent finding in diffuse fatty infiltration. These different patterns of fat deposition can sometimes mimic neoplastic conditions, leading to unnecessary diagnostic tests, and invasive procedures. This can be avoided by the assessment of fat content, location, contrast enhancement, mass effect, and morphology of the affected area. Imaging modalities like sonoelastography, CT, and MRI are the front runners in quantification of hepatic steatosis and may minimise the need for invasive procedures. Specificity and sensitivity for the detection of fatty liver deposition have been reported to range between 60-100% (77%-95% for US, 43%-95% for unenhanced CT, and 81% and 100% for chemical shift GRE MR imaging). For the assessment of intralesional fat chemical shift GRE is the most reliable. US, CT, and MRI may be unreliable if the fat content is less than 30%. Newer MRI sequences under development will be more sensitive than current ones in use today.

CONFLICT OF INTEREST

The authors confirm that they have no conflict of interest to declare for this publication.

ACKNOWLEDGEMENTS

Declared none.

REFERENCES

[1]   Sanyal AJ. Nonalcoholic steatohepatitis. Clin Perspect Gastroenterol 2000; 5: 129-39.

[2]   Joseph AE, Saverymuttu SH, al-Sam S, Cook MG, Maxwell JD. Comparison of liver histology with ultrasonography in assessing diffuse parenchymal liver disease. Clin Radiol 1991; 43(1): 26-31.
[http://dx.doi.org/10.1016/S0009-9260(05)80350-2] [PMID: 1999069]

[3]   Webb M, Yeshua H, Zelber-Sagi S, *et al.* Diagnostic value of a computerized hepatorenal index for sonographic quantification of liver steatosis. AJR Am J Roentgenol 2009; 192(4): 909-14.
[http://dx.doi.org/10.2214/AJR.07.4016] [PMID: 19304694]

[4]   Yoneda M, Suzuki K, Kato S, *et al.* Nonalcoholic fatty liver disease: US-based acoustic radiation force impulse elastography. Radiology 2010; 256(2): 640-7.
[http://dx.doi.org/10.1148/radiol.10091662] [PMID: 20529989]

[5]   Saadeh S, Younossi ZM, Remer EM, *et al.* The utility of radiological imaging in nonalcoholic fatty liver disease. Gastroenterology 2002; 123(3): 745-50.
[http://dx.doi.org/10.1053/gast.2002.35354] [PMID: 12198701]

[6]   Shigefuku R, Takahashi H, Kato M, *et al.* Evaluation of hepatic tissue blood flow using xenon computed tomography with fibrosis progression in nonalcoholic fatty liver disease: comparison with chronic hepatitis C. Int J Mol Sci 2014; 15(1): 1026-39.
[http://dx.doi.org/10.3390/ijms15011026] [PMID: 24424317]

[7]   Singh D, Das CJ, Baruah MP. Imaging of non alcoholic fatty liver disease: A road less travelled. Indian J Endocrinol Metab 2013; 17(6): 990-5.
[http://dx.doi.org/10.4103/2230-8210.122606] [PMID: 24381873]

[8]   van Werven JR, Marsman HA, Nederveen AJ, *et al.* Assessment of hepatic steatosis in patients undergoing liver resection: comparison of US, CT, T1-weighted dual-echo MR imaging, and point-resolved 1H MR spectroscopy. Radiology 2010; 256(1): 159-68.
[http://dx.doi.org/10.1148/radiol.10091790] [PMID: 20574093]

[9]   Loomba R, Wolfson T, Ang B, *et al.* Magnetic resonance elastography predicts advanced fibrosis in patients with nonalcoholic fatty liver disease: a prospective study. Hepatology 2014; 60(6): 1920-8.
[http://dx.doi.org/10.1002/hep.27362] [PMID: 25103310]

CHAPTER 4

Histopathological Changes of NAFLD

Peter Nagy[*]

Department of Pathology and Experimental Cancer Research, Semmelweis University, Budapest, Hungary

Abstract: Nonalcoholic fatty liver disease (NAFLD) is one of the most common chronic liver diseases worldwide. Although imaging techniques and serologic testing are important examinations, histology remains the gold standard to establish the diagnosis, to stratify to grade and stage the actual sample. There are two major subtypes of NAFLD, simple steatosis and the progressive form nonalcoholic steatohepatitis (NASH). Simple steatosis is characterized by fat accumulation in hepatocytes. NASH can be diagnosed if, in addition to steatosis, inflammation and hepatocyte damage in the form of ballooning is present in the liver. There may be other histological alterations with variable significance *e.g.* fibrosis, ductular reaction, granulomas, Mallory-Denk bodies, *etc.* NASH is a progressive disease, which can end up in cirrhosis. Hepatocellular carcinoma (HCC) is also a well-known complication of NASH. It can develop in cirrhotic and surprisingly in non-cirrhotic stage of NASH. The histological signs of NASH can be substantially different in pediatric patients, than in adults. Several histological scoring systems have been developed for reliable grading and staging of NAFLD. They can be used to follow up the progression of the disease, monitor the efficacy of potential therapies and to compare different studies. Future will decide which one of them proves to be most reliable, and reproducible. Finally, histological diagnosis can be important to distinguish NAFLD from other chronic liver diseases or recognize comorbidities.

Keywords: Ballooning, Cirrhosis, Ductular reaction, Hepatic fibrosis, Hepatocellular carcinoma, Mallory-Denk bodies, Scoring, Steatohepatitis, Steatosis.

INTRODUCTION

Non-alcoholic fatty liver disease (NAFLD) is the most common cause of chronically elevated levels of serum alanine transaminase (ALT) in both Western and developing societies. It is more common than viral hepatitis or alcoholic liver disease. Its exact prevalence is not known, however an estimated nearly 30% of

[*] **Corresponding author Peter Nagy:** Department of Pathology and Experimental Cancer Research, Semmelweis University, Budapest, Hungary; Tel:36-1-317 1074; E-mail: pdrnagy@gmail.com

Tatjana Ábel & Gabriella Lengyel (Eds.)
All rights reserved-© 2017 Bentham Science Publishers

the population is affected in the USA, UK or China, and it is more frequently diagnosed in children [1]. Therefore, it represents an enormous health care issue requiring further efforts to develop new strategies for its prevention and treatment.

NAFLD is defined as increased accumulation of hepatic triglyceride, steatosis, without excess alcohol consumption (<20g/day for men, <10g/day for women). It is the hepatic manifestation of metabolic syndrome and can be considered as a consequence of systemic and hepatic insulin resistance. NAFLD can manifest as a broad range of histological changes, from simple steatosis to non-alcoholic steatohepatitis (NASH). This latter form can progress into liver cirrhosis and NAFLD is more often thought to serve as a basis for the development of hepatocellular carcinoma (HCC) in cirrhotic or non-cirrhotic liver. Not only liver diseases and mortality are more common in people with NAFLD, recent epidemiologic studies indicate that cardiovascular diseases and non-hepatic forms of cancer are more common in patients with simple steatosis, while steatosis and diabetes or NASH are important risk factors for liver-related mortality [2]. Seventy per cent of centrally obese patients with hypertension and diabetes have steatohepatitis shown by liver biopsy [3]. An early diagnosis of the affected individuals is extremely important. NASH is usually considered as a condition, which is preceded by simple steatosis and insulin resistance. However, there are evidences suggesting that NASH and simple steatosis could arise as two independent alterations. This is supported by the fact that progression of steatosis into NASH is rarely observed. . Although steatosis and NASH are still considered as histological subtypes along the spectrum of NAFLD, they are likely different entities not only from histological but also from pathophysiological standpoint. The most widely used and simplest screening laboratory test for liver dysfunction is the determination of serum ALT level. This examination, however, has proven to be very unreliable in recognizing patients with NAFLD. In several well-documented studies, normal ALT levels were found even in advanced stages of the disease. In 40% of the children with varying degree of fibrosis, the ALT value was in the normal range and almost 10% of adults with NAFLD-related cirrhosis had no elevated transaminase level [4].

Imaging techniques can provide a significant help in recognizing NAFLD patients, but they are really efficient only in patients with an advanced disease when the fat content is increased in more than 33% of the hepatocytes [5]. Unfortunately, there is no available simple blood test or imaging technique that could differentiate simple steatosis from NASH. The simplest and cheapest technology, ultrasound, shows a high level of interobserver variability. The most reliable magnetic resonance imaging (MRI) is very expensive and it is not available for screening examinations [6]. The combination of serologic and imaging markers and associated clinical algorithms has advanced to a great extent in the last few years, but still cannot replace the histological examination of liver samples, which despite its limitations remains the "gold standard" for confirming or excluding NASH in suspicious patients.

GENERAL HISTOLOGICAL FEATURES OF NAFLD

The hallmark of NAFLD is the hepatocellular steatosis or fatty change. Fatty hepatocytes may occur occasionally in normal liver, but the presence of fat in more than 5% of the hepatocytes is regarded as pathological. The NAFLD-associated fatty change is usually macrovesicular, but microvesicular form may also develop sometimes. The fatty hepatocytes appear first around the central veins in zone 3 of the hepatic acinus (Fig. **1**), but the whole lobule may be involved, depending on the severity of the process.

The severity of steatosis is usually divided into 3 categories: mild (5-33%), moderate (33-66%), and severe (>66%). The extent of steatosis shows some correlation with the activity of inflammation; patients with severe fatty changes are more likely to have NASH.

The major histopathological components of steatohepatitis are: steatosis, inflammation (lobular and portal) and the so called ballooning of hepatocytes, a morphological sign of hepatocyte damage (Table **1**).

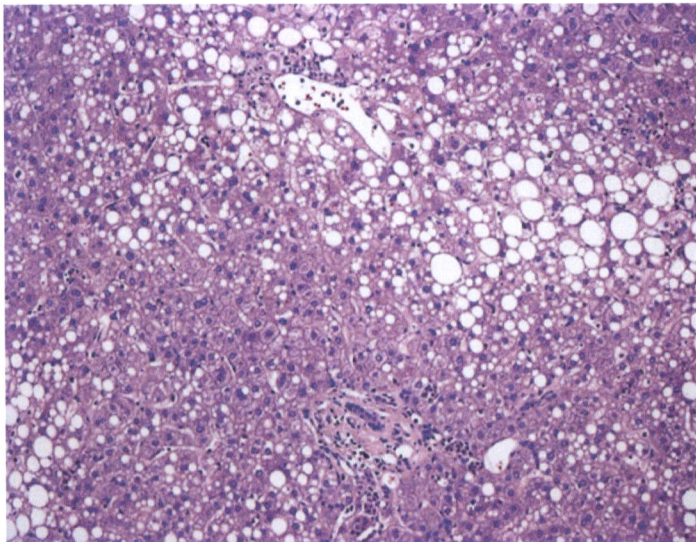

Fig. (1). The hallmark of NAFLD is fatty change. The steatotic hepatocytes have preferential pericentral (zone 3) distribution.

Table 1. Correlation between the most important morphological features of NAFLD.

	Macroves steatosis	Microves steatosis	Lobular inflammation	Portal inflammation	Cent fibrosis	Port fibrosis	Ballooning	MDB	Ductular reaction
Macroves steatosis	Ø	+	-	-	-	-	-	-	-
Microves steatosis	+	Ø	-	-	+	-	+	+	-
Lobular inflammation	-	-	Ø	-	+	-	+	+	-
Portal inflammation	-	-	-	Ø	-	+	-	-	+
Cent fibrosis	-	+	+	-	Ø	-	+	+	-
Port fibrosis	-	-	-	+	-	Ø	-	-	+
Ballooning	-	+	+	-	+	-	Ø	+	-
MDB	-	+	+	-	+	-	+	Ø	-
Ductular reaction	-	-	-	+	-	+	-	-	Ø

These are the minimal criteria for the diagnosis of adult NASH; other lesions like fibrosis, ductular proliferation might be present but they are not required. All these changes are usually more advanced in the perivenular zone [7, 8].

The lobular component of the inflammation is usually more prominent than the portal one in the common form of adult NASH. It is usually characterized by a mixed inflammatory cell infiltrate dominated by mononuclear cells. Enlargement and aggregation of Kupffer cells can also be seen around the terminal hepatic venules. Microgranulomas or even larger lipogranulomas are formed in some liver samples. Sometimes the ballooned hepatocytes are surrounded by neutrophil granulocytes; this process is called "satellitosis", its presence in a high number raises the suspicion of alcoholic liver disease (ALD). Mononuclear cells are typically predominant in the portal component of the inflammation. Advanced portal inflammation in NASH is associated with increased steatosis, ballooning and fibrosis. In case of very intense portal inflammation and formation of lymphoid follicles, concerns for concomitant liver diseases *e.g.* hepatitis C infection or autoimmune hepatitis can be raised [9].

Hepatocellular injury may also be present in NASH in the form of apoptotic bodies, lytic necrosis; however, the most typical form is ballooning. Ballooned hepatocytes are enlarged with rarefied, reticular cytoplasm. Cytoplasmic aggregates referred to as Mallory-Denk bodies (MDB) may be present in them, similarly fat droplets can be seen occasionally in these cells. Ballooned hepatocytes are most frequently seen in the perivenular zone and if fibrosis is present, they are commonly surrounded by perisinusoidal collagen fibers [10].

In adult NASH, initially the fibrosis is located in zone 3 in the perisinusoidal spaces; it is commonly described as pericellular (chickenwire). Fibrosis is usually associated with active inflammation but it may also be present in simple steatosis, probably indicating a preexistent episode of NASH. With the progression of disease, the fibrotic bundles become denser and later portal and periportal deposition of collagen also become obvious and may result in the complete reconstruction of the hepatic structure, the formation of cirrhosis. At this stage, the steatosis may disappear; NASH-related cirrhosis is usually macronodular or mixed [11].

Additional histological alterations may be present in NASH. The emergence of ductular structures in the portal zone represents the activation of hepatic stem/progenitor cell compartment and is usually referred to as ductular reaction [12, 13]. Mild hemosiderosis may be hepatocellular, sinusoidal or both. At present it is not clear if iron accumulation alters the outcome of the disease. Hepatocytes may contain large eosinophilic cytoplasmic inclusions; these are enlarged mitochondria and are called megamitochondria. They can be recognized by light microscope; electron microscopy can reveal paracrystalline inclusions and loss of cristae. The importance of these lesions is not clear. They probably reflect injury from lipid peroxidation or adaptive changes [14]. Vacuolated nuclei preferentially in periportal hepatocytes may derive from glycogen deposition in nuclei. Since this lesion is thought to be very rare in ALD, it may be useful for the distinction of NASH from ALD-related steatohepatitis [9].

THE ROLE AND VALUE OF LIVER BIOPSY IN THE DIAGNOSIS AND TREATMENT OF NAFLD PATIENTS

Although there have been enormous advancements in the imaging and serologic testing of liver diseases including NAFLD, they are still not able to replace histological examination of the liver tissue [11]. However, liver biopsy is an expensive, even more, invasive procedure, not without rare but potentially dangerous complications for the patients, thus liver biopsy cannot be applied as a screening examination. It must address well-defined questions. It would be a mistake to consider non-invasive tests and biopsy on an either/or basis. It could be one of the important purposes to perform non-invasive examinations to identify those patients for whom histological examination may provide more benefits. The potential complications of taking histological samples from the liver include minor pain, perforation/injury for other organs; bleeding has been reported in

0.3% of the cases and even death of the patients has occurred at 0.01% [15]. If such a risk is taken, one should gain maximum information from the sample. However, adequate analysis can be performed only on appropriate specimen. Wedge biopsy is not suitable for such examination, since the subcapsular layer of the liver is more fibrotic, and samples from such location may be misleading. The size of the biopsy sample is also critical. Liver tissue taken by a narrow-bore needle may contain only transected portal areas, and these samples are not acceptable for the evaluation of parenchymal liver disease. It is recommended that the length of the specimen should be at least 1.6cm with a diameter of 1.2-1.8mm, and it should contain 10 portal fields at least [9, 11]. Although some studies have described moderate histologic variability between lobes *e.g.* there may be smaller portal areas in the right lobe than in the left, the location is usually not critical. These "fine-tuning" of sampling should be considered in systematic, comparative studies or in case of repeated biopsies during follow-up of patients. In the everyday routine practice, the experience of the pathologist is more critical for the correct evaluation of the sample. There are unavoidable interobserver disagreements on the extent of steatosis, fibrosis, ballooning and other parameters. The concordance between the reports can be increased, as in any other fields of pathology, if the liver biopsies are evaluated by experienced, specially trained hepatic pathologists.

Liver biopsy is taken usually from patients suspected to have NAFLD, but the non-invasive tests have not provided an unambiguous diagnosis. In these cases, the most important task for the biopsy is to confirm or exclude the diagnosis. In large comparative studies, usually 30% of the patients had something other than NAFLD [16]. Association of NAFLD with other liver diseases can be also diagnosed by liver biopsy [9]. It is not rare that patients who have serologically diagnosed viral hepatitis show histological signs of fatty liver disease; it also can be recognized in patients who are routinely biopsied for autoimmune hepatitis or primary biliary cirrhosis. Histological examinations are recommended for morbidly obese patients who are going to undergo bariatric surgery. NASH and/or cirrhosis have been diagnosed in 25% and 3% of the patients respectively and this has major impact on further therapeutic decisions [17]. Biopsy is the most adequate or in fact the only adequate way to stratify NAFLD patients. Simple steatosis can only be reliably distinguished from steatohepatitis by histological examination [18]. While the former is a non-progressive disease and these patients are usually not at increased risk of mortality attributable to liver diseases compared to the average population, the latter carries an increased risk for progression. The severity of NAFLD can be characterized by different histological scoring systems [7]. This kind of examination provides the only reliable diagnosis about the rate of progression, efficiency of therapeutic intervention, *etc*.

Liver biopsies contributed a lot to our understanding of the mechanism of NAFLD and provided valuable epidemiologic data. Nowadays, the majority of cryptogenic cirrhotic cases are considered as burned out NAFLD-related liver diseases. This connection was revealed by histological examinations [19]. The association of increased probability of cardiovascular diseases with NAFLD was recognized by performing liver biopsies on obese children who had or had not NAFLD [20].

The 2012 guidelines from the American Association for the Study of Liver Disease (AASLD) state that liver biopsy should be reserved for subjects who will "benefit", for subjects with potentially competing diagnoses, and for children with either an unclear diagnosis or in whom consideration is being given to medication [21]. In addition, the European Association for the Study of Liver Diseases (EASLD) recommends biopsies in all bariatric surgery candidates and as an endpoint in all clinical trials. Liver biopsy should be offered to patients with higher risk for advanced disease such as old age, obesity, diabetes and/or elevated ALT values after 6 months of diet, exercise and other treatments for metabolic syndrome [22]. A recent decision analysis study comparing the long-term benefit of biopsy *vs.* no biopsy decision in NAFLD patients concluded that early diagnosis and treatment by means of liver biopsy resulted in milder process, slower progression, and less patients who required liver transplantation [23]. In addition, there was a survival advantage in the biopsied patients even if the risk of biopsy-related death was included. Histopathological evaluation of liver biopsies provides unsurpassed information about the form, grade and stage of the actual NAFLD disease and remains central to all investigations, and thus histological changes are in the focus of the following pages.

HISTOLOGICAL CHARACTERISTICS OF NAFLD

Steatosis

Steatosis or fatty change is the most important histological lesion of NAFLD; in fact the name of the syndrome derives from hepatic fat accumulation. Fat droplets in hepatocytes are physiological in certain species *e.g.* migrating birds but the normal human liver contains no visible fat. Day and James [24] proposed the original "two hit" hypothesis as a mechanism of NASH. The accumulation of fat would be the primary event, followed by an oxidative injury and subsequent necro-inflammation. Recently, systemic lipotoxicity is the most accepted explanation for the development of NASH [25], when excess or dysregulation of free fatty acids (FFA) is the triggering event. This theory links overnutrition, dietary changes and dysfunctional lipid distribution to insulin resistance, which eventually causes cellular injury. According to this theory, fat accumulation in hepatocytes is a consequence of excess FFA, and therefore it can be regarded as a protective mechanism, sequestering toxic FFA in the form of triglycerides. The primary sources of hepatic FFA are triglyceride lipolysis in adipocytes and "*de novo*" lipogenesis in hepatocytes. The contribution of dietary fat is moderate. Circulatory triglycerides are not a direct source of fat in hepatocytes, a reduction of serum triglyceride level exerts no significant beneficial effect on the liver. However, patients with NASH have highly elevated serum FFA after a fatty meal, indicating the importance of individual metabolic pathways. There is a well-known connection between overnutrition, metabolic syndrome and NAFLD; the connection is even closer with the amount of visceral fat and insulin resistance [26]. Experimental results indicate that triglyceride accumulation *per se* is not harmful to hepatocytes and may even represent a protective mechanism against lipotoxicity. However, other types of lipid, *e.g.* free fatty acids and free cholesterol are linked to hepatocellular damage, inflammation and progression into steatohepatitis. Unfortunately, the different types of lipids cannot be distinguished histologically. It seems that lipid compartmentalization and especially the ratio of monounsaturated and saturated free fatty acids are the important determinants of the development of either simple steatosis or progressive steatohepatitis and fibrosis. These observations indicate that the most important roles in disease progression in NAFLD are played by the quality and not the quantity of lipids accumulating in the liver [27].

The fat is lost from tissues during traditional histologic processing. Thus, fat usually presents in the form of an empty vacuole on hematoxylin and eosin (H&E) stained sections made from paraffin-embedded tissue. If there is any doubt about the origin of the vacuoles, fat staining can confirm the suspicion but it must be performed on frozen sections.

The histological criterion of NAFLD is the presence of fat droplets (empty vacuoles) in more than 5% of the hepatocytes. There are two different forms of fatty changes in the liver with different clinical implications: macro- and microvesicular steatosis.

The macrovesicular form of steatosis is more common. In this case, there is a single, large fat droplet in the hepatocyte displacing the other cytoplasmic components and the nucleus; these hepatocytes look like adipocytes (Fig. **2**).

Sometimes there are more, smaller but well-circumscribed droplets in the cytoplasm; this is a variant of macrovesicular steatosis referred to as "small droplet" steatosis (Fig. **3**), it should not be confused with microvesicular fatty change. Small droplets are often present around larger ones and may fuse to form macrodroplets.

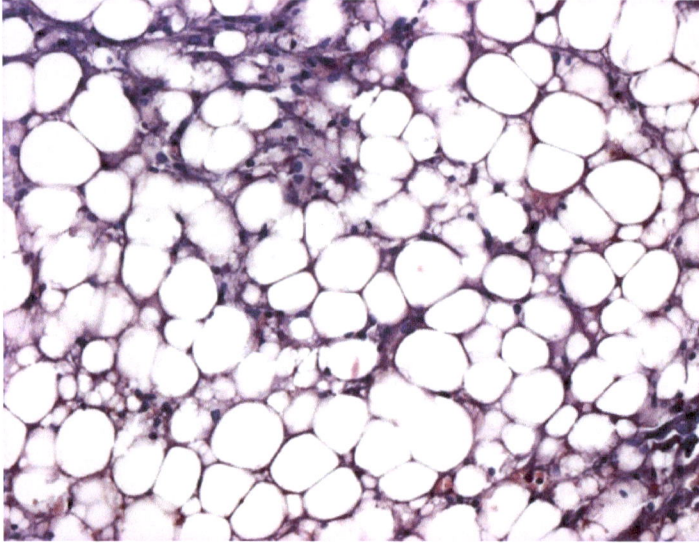

Fig. (2). Severe macrovesicular steatosis, the hepatocytes look like adipocytes.

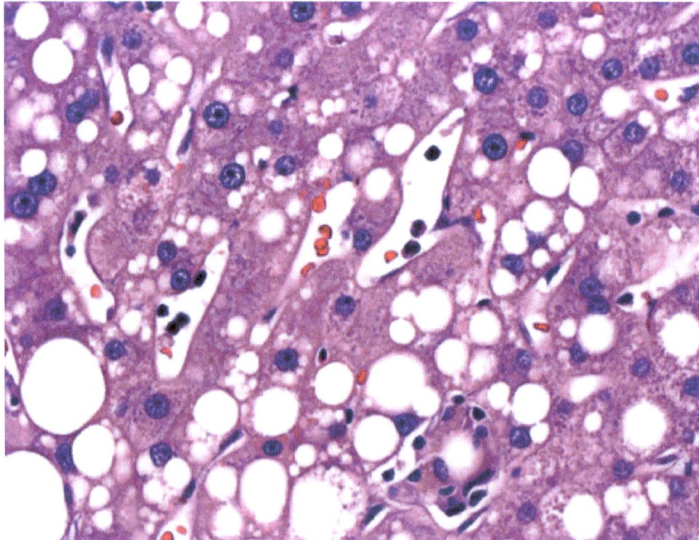

Fig. (3). Mixed form of macrovesicular steatosis, "small droplets" are present beside the large fat vacuoles.

Macrovesicular steatosis appears first in the pericentral zone (zone 3), because this part of the hepatic lobule is at the largest distance from the terminal branches of portal vein and hepatic arteries, providing blood rich in oxygen and nutrients for the hepatic parenchyma. Steatosis can be panacinar in severe cases, or its distribution may be irregular "azonal" when resolving. The severity of steatosis is usually classified into 3 grades as described earlier. Immunohistochemical studies have shown differential expression of lipid-droplet-associated proteins perilipin 1 and perilipin 2 (adipophilin) but no alterations of perilipin 3 expression [28, 29]. The significance of these changes is still debated.

The other form, the so-called microvesicular steatosis is characterized by distended hepatocytes with tiny lipid droplets (less than 1 μm in diameter) (Fig. **4**). The nucleus remains centrally located, differently from macrovesicular steatosis, where it is pushed to the periphery. Since the small lipid vesicles may not be discernible, special fat staining *e.g.* oil red O may be required to confirm the diagnosis. Diffuse forms of microvesicular steatosis occur in Reye syndrome or in acute fatty liver of pregnancy.

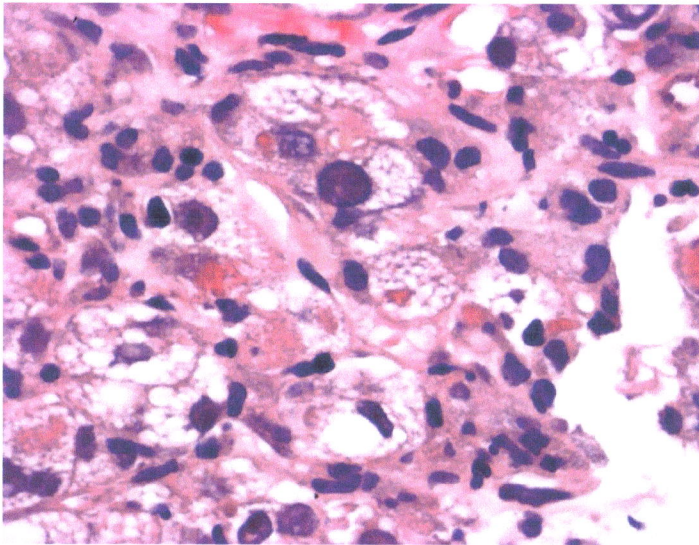

Fig. (4). Focal microvesicular steatosis.

These diseases are the consequences of severe mitochondrial β-oxidation defects due to genetic or acquired causes. They are special clinical entities completely separate from NAFLD, and are often associated with hepatic encephalopathy and liver failure. These syndromes can be lethal or may resolve but do not progress into chronic disease as NAFLD. Microvesicular steatosis is present up to 10% of liver biopsies in patients with NAFLD. It usually occurs in clusters of hepatocytes showing an azonal distribution pattern. The microvesicular fatty change is associated with more severe macrovesicular steatosis, hepatocyte ballooning, more advanced fibrosis, higher NAS scores and with the presence of Mallory-Denk bodies (MDB) and megamitochondria, that is with histological hallmarks of hepatocyte injury and cytoskeletal damage [30]. The extent of macrovesicular steatosis can decrease with the advance of disease, while the microvesicular form may even progress. Thus, the presence of microvesicular steatosis in liver biopsy may indicate a severe, progressive form of NASH.

Steatosis is present in all forms of NAFLD but serial biopsies in patients with NASH have confirmed that the degree of fatty change decreases in livers with progression and it can completely disappear in some burn-out cirrhosis. Pathologists should carefully apply the diagnosis of "steatosis" or "fatty change", since simple steatosis is usually a non-progressive form of NAFLD. If other histopathological lesions indicating cellular injury and consequent inflammatory response are associated, this should be emphasized in the pathological report.

Inflammation

Inflammation is another basic histological component of NAFLD, which must be evaluated carefully, because it has serious clinical implications. Longitudinal studies have proven that the presence of inflammation is an independent predictor of advanced fibrosis, demonstrating its significance in the pathogenesis of progressive NASH [10]. There are two separable forms of inflammatory reactions in NAFLD. Lobular inflammation is an essential component of NASH; in fact it must be present for establishing the diagnosis. The presence of portal inflammation is not absolutely necessary for the diagnosis, but it is also an important prognostic factor.

The lobular inflammatory reaction is usually mild and it is more dominant in the perivenular zone (zone 3). It consists of both acute and chronic inflammatory cells. The parenchymal inflammation can be quantitated by the number of necro-inflammatory foci in a 20-fold magnified optical field. Neutrophil granulocytes occur mostly within the sinusoid, ballooned hepatocytes with MDB-s are sometimes surrounded by polymorphonuclears. This lesion, called satellitosis is explained by the chemotactic feature of MDBs. Eosinophils are usually in the neighborhood of lipogranulomas. Chronic inflammatory cells are mostly CD3+ T lymphocytes, plasma cells and hepatic macrophages, Kupffer cells. Lipogranulomas are special structures characteristic to lobular steatohepatitis. They consist of rare eosinophils, Kupffer cells, and mononuclears surrounding steatotic hepatocytes or large fat droplets. They are also more common in the pericentral zone, but they can occur anywhere in the hepatic lobule or sometimes even in the portal space. They are commonly associated with the presence of fibrosis. The demonstration of Kupffer cells with diastase-resistant PAS-positive cytoplasmic granules refers to preceding necro-inflammatory reaction in the liver. The Kupffer cells are relatively evenly distributed in normal or in uncomplicated fatty liver, while they are concentrated in the perivenular zone in steatohepatitis. The number of Kupffer cells correlates with necro-inflammatory activity and the stage of fibrosis [31]. Therefore, the macrophages are thought to play an important role in the progression of NASH by inducing fibrosis with TGFβ secretion, contributing to hepatocyte injury and regulating other aspects of the inflammatory reaction. Experimental data, however, indicate that macrophages can also participate in the degradation of different extracellular matrix components and contribute to the regression of fibrosis [32].

Portal inflammatory reaction in NAFLD is less characterized, it is more common in children, but interestingly in both adults and children, lobular or acinar inflammatory scores have no association with those of the extent of portal inflammation [33]. In fact, increased portal inflammation has been described with advanced fibrosis, while it is well known that as fibrosis progresses, steatosis and the activity of lobular inflammation regress, and it may be completely lacking from the resulting cirrhosis. The portal inflammation in NAFLD is usually mild and consists of mostly lymphocytes. Interestingly, the number of portal macrophages is consistently elevated in simple steatosis, which is considered a benign disease. The early accumulation of macrophages supports an initiating role of the innate immune system in NAFLD. Natural killer (NK) T cells, which are present in the normal liver, but mostly disappear during simple steatosis, reappear again in steatohepatitis [34]. The presence of "more than mild" portal inflammation in adults is not associated with autoantibodies and elevated ALT level, but it is associated with older age, female gender, and higher body mass index, elevated insulin levels, with coexistent diabetes and hypertension and surprisingly with medications for NAFLD [33]. The extent of portal but not lobular inflammation is significantly associated with the intensity of periportal ductular reaction [35]. Previous observations have also suggested that increased portal inflammation in untreated NAFLD patients was a reliable marker of advanced disease, but in treated patients, irrespective of the type of therapy, it was considered as a sign of disease resolution [36].

Hepatocellular Injury, Ballooning

The third required component of steatohepatitis is hepatocellular injury represented by apoptosis, lytic necrosis and ballooning [37]. Acidophilic bodies, also referred to as Councilman bodies, are apoptotic hepatocytes. They are present only shortly in the hepatic tissue because they are phagocytosed quickly and disappear. Thus, their counting usually results in an underestimation of apoptotic activity. Increased apoptosis rate in NASH is supported by histopathological studies on clinical samples and experimental animal models. Sensitive and reliable apoptosis detection techniques, such as TUNEL test or immunohistochemical detection of caspases 3 and 7, demonstrate apoptotic cells significantly more often in NASH samples than in simple steatosis or in normal liver tissue. Even more positive correlation is found between apoptosis rate and AST/ALT ratio, inflammation activity and the stage of fibrosis [38]. Both the extrinsic (CD95/Fas) and the intrinsic (Noxa) apoptosis pathways are activated and correlate with the serum FFA level. Fas receptor and TNF receptor I are upregulated in human NASH livers and the serum FFA level are thought to be responsible for the increased expression, but the TNF level is also higher in these patients providing rational explanation for the increased rate of apoptosis [39]. Endoplasmic reticulum stress can also contribute to the induction of apoptosis and it is considered to be a cause as well as a consequence of steatohepatitis [40]. Increased ER stress marker expression is also characteristic of NAFLD and genetic manipulation of mice inhibiting ER stress also makes the experimental animals more resistant to steatosis. Autophagy dysregulation has been also suggested to contribute to the pathogenesis of NAFLD [41].

Hepatocellular ballooning is a unique form of hepatocellular injury. Ballooned hepatocytes are large (usually have a diameter more, than 30µm), round, and have pale staining reticulated cytoplasm (Fig. **5**). They are common in alcoholic and non-alcoholic steatohepatitis, but they can be seen in other liver diseases as Wilson's disease, chronic cholestasis, or allograft rejection. Like other typical NASH lesions ballooned hepatocytes are more common in the perivenular zone in the neighborhood of steatotic hepatocytes. They might have small fat droplets in their cytoplasm. It is also very characteristic of these hepatocytes that immunohistochemically detectable K8/18 expression is missing [42]. Combination of oil red O staining with K18 immunostaining proved to be a very reliable way of detecting ballooned hepatocytes. This might be important considering that the presence of ballooned hepatocytes is required for establishing the diagnosis of NASH, and the interobserver disagreement is the highest in the recognition of these cells. Perilipin/ADRP/TIP47 protein expression changes have also been described in ballooned hepatocytes [43]. It is hypothesized that the disposal of FFA, lipid accumulation in ER can result in further oxidative stress and dilatation of ER in these cells. Ballooning is a key feature for the distinction of progressive steatohepatitis from simple steatosis.

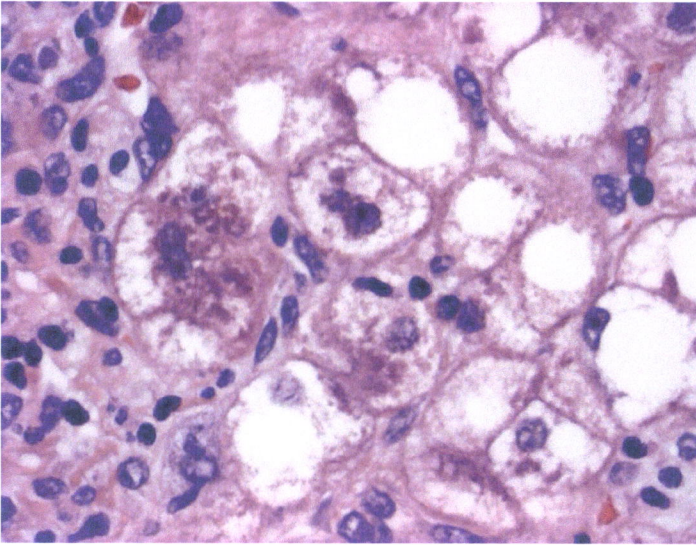

Fig. (5). Ballooning, large round hepatocytes with reticulated cytoplasm, occasional fat droplets.

Ballooned hepatocytes may or may not contain another typical lesion of NASH, Mallory-Denk bodies (Fig. **6**). These structures were first described in the early nineteenth century by Mallory as hyaline inclusion bodies in alcoholic liver disease [44] and have been referred to as Mallory or alcoholic hyaline. They have been recently renamed to acknowledge the contribution of Helmut Denk to the understanding of their formation. In addition to NASH, they are present in several other liver diseases such as ALD, Wilson's disease, chronic cholestasis, focal nodular hyperplasia, hepatocellular adenoma or carcinoma. MDBs are protein aggregates consisting of K8/K18, ubiquitin and p62 [45]. MDBs ultrastructurally are constructed by 5-20nm thick filaments either arranged in parallel (type I) or randomly oriented (type II); type III MDBs also contain amorphous, granular material [45]. MDBs can be easily recognized on hematoxylin and eosin stained sections, they are present approximately in a third of NASH liver biopsies.

Immunostaining for K8/K18 is a more sensitive method, which can visualize milder alterations of K8/K18 network, but this is usually not required in everyday routine examinations. MDBs are always found in ballooned hepatocytes, they can vary in size from tiny little cytoplasmic granules to large cytoplasmic inclusions. The presence of MDBs can help to identify ballooned hepatocytes, thus they are important diagnostic markers, but their prognostic value in NASH is still debated. While they are strongly associated with ballooned hepatocytes, an indicator of severe disease, no correlation was found between the presence of MDBs and the severity of NASH. The mechanism of MDB formation is also not clear. While a misbalance between protein folding, repair and degradation seems to be important, direct connection between MDB formation and oxidative stress is missing [46]. MDBs represent one of the most abundant inclusion bodies in human tissues, but their exact role is obscure like other similar structures in Alzheimer's and Parkinson's disease.

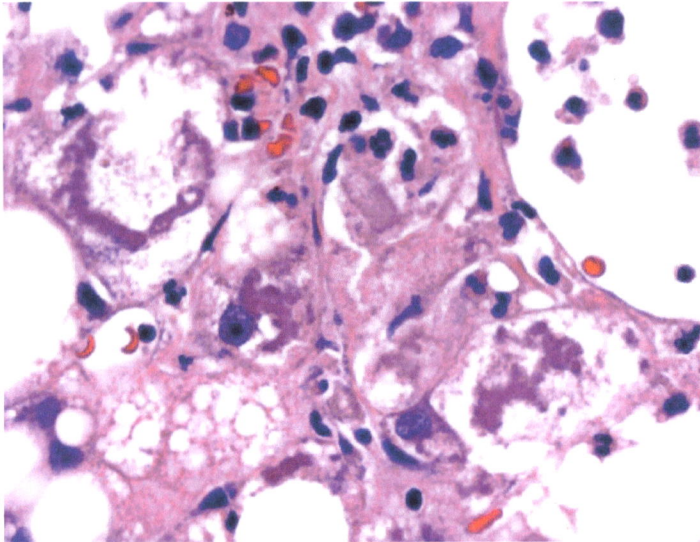

Fig. (6). Mallory-Denk bodies, irregular, granular cytoplasmic inclusions in ballooned hepatocytes.

Liver Fibrosis and Ductular Reaction

Liver fibrosis is the final common pathway of practically all sorts of chronic hepatic injuries, NAFLD is not exempted. Two different patterns of liver fibrosis: perivenular and periportal can be clearly distinguished in NAFLD [8]. Interestingly, the distribution of fibrosis depends on the age of the patients. Centrilobular dominance of fibrosis is typical in adults, while NAFLD in children is mostly characterized by pure periportal fibrosis, accompanied by periportal steatosis and inflammation. However, portal fibrosis and progressing periportal septa can be present in adult patients as well. In the liver, activated hepatic stellate cells (HSC) are the major sources of the deposited extracellular matrix material, including type I and III collagens [13]. Hepatic stellate cells reside in the perisinusoidal space of Disse. Under normal circumstances, HSCs are quiescent and contain droplets of vitamin A, explaining their other name, fat storing cells. Upon different kinds of liver injury, HSCs transdifferentiate into activated myofibroblasts. They lose vitamin A, start to express smooth muscle actin, desmin and gain contractility. All sorts of inflammatory cells, Kupffer cells, platelets, damaged hepatocytes are the sources of platelet-derived growth factor (PDGF) and transforming growth factor beta (TGF-β), the two growth factors, which are mostly responsible for the activation of HSCs. In case of NASH, lipotoxicity is proposed to be the major mechanism triggering fibrogenesis. In typical adult NASH, this occurs in the perivenular zone, at the site of hepatocellular injury resulting in the peculiar pericellular, "chicken wire" fibrosis. In pediatric NASH, and often in adult patients also portal fibrosis develops despite the dominant lobular hepatocellular injury [47]. The two different patterns of fibrosis suggest the presence of alternative fibrogenic pathways in NASH.

Peculiar bile duct-like structures referred to as ductular reaction [48] often develop periportally in chronic liver diseases (Fig. **7**). These ductules are the extensions of canals of Hering, the smallest branches of intrahepatic biliary tree.

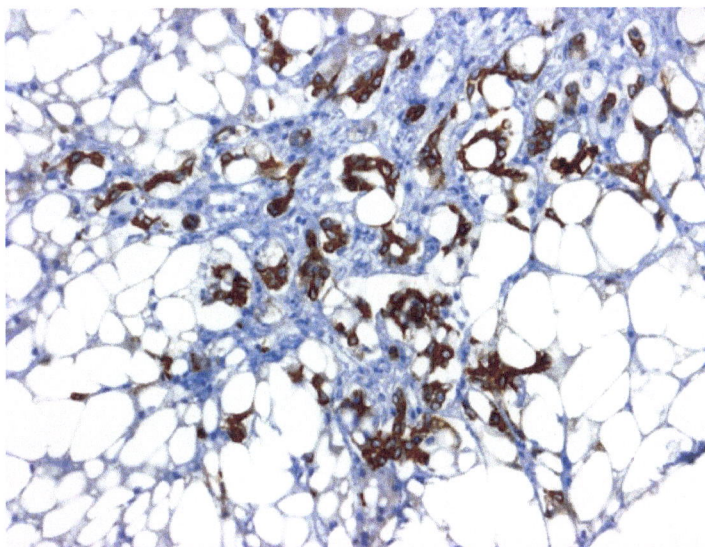

Fig. (7). Ductular reaction. Cytokeratin 7 immunostaining outlines the proliferating ductules in the periportal zone.

The hepatic progenitor/stem cells are residing in the canals of Hering; therefore cells constructing the ductular reaction are thought to be the progenies of hepatic stem/progenitor cells. The hepatic stem cells are facultative stem cells because they are silent under normal circumstances and do not contribute to the everyday cell turnover. Even after severe injuries, the hepatocytes are able to return into the cell cycle and regenerate the hepatic parenchyma. The hepatic stem cells represent a backup compartment, which is activated only when the hepatocytes are compromised due to some chronic injury and are no more able to regenerate efficiently. The presence of ductular reaction indicates such regenerative effort of the hepatic stem cell compartment. The regenerative role of ductular reaction is proven by the appearance of intermediate hepatocytes (Fig. **8**), which are transitional forms between progenitor cells and hepatocytes. Hepatic myofibroblasts are always present in close proximity with the ductular reaction because they are regarded as an important component of the special microenvironment around progenitor cells, also called "niche". In case of NASH, the prolonged oxidative stress inhibits the regenerative capacity of hepatocytes leading to the compensatory expansion of progenitor cells in the form of ductular reaction [13].

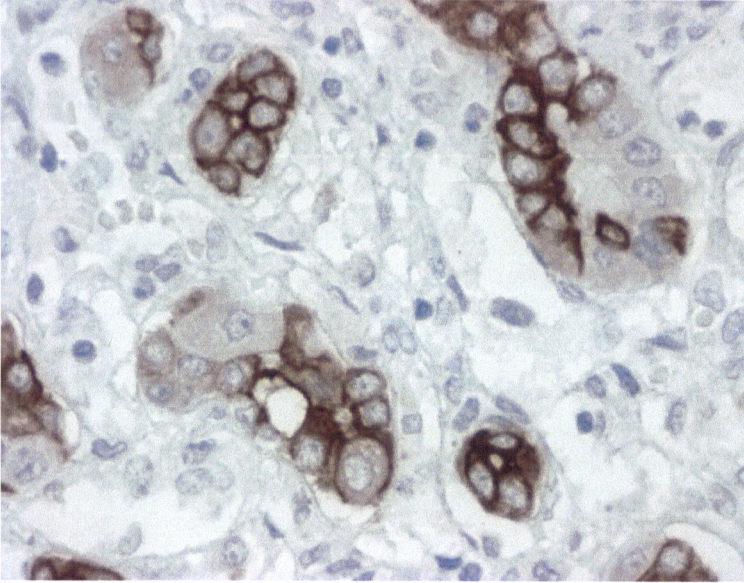

Fig. (8). Intermediary hepatobiliary cells. Cytokeratin 7 immunostaining decorates the ductules, which contain scattered enlarged cells. The fading of CK7 staining indicates the hepatocytic differentiation.

It has been proven that ductular reaction strongly and independently correlates with progressive periportal fibrosis. In fact, ductular reaction is a major pathway, which drives hepatic fibrosis in NASH causing the progressive periportal fibrosis. This is supported by observations showing that the expansion of ductular reaction is correlated with the extent of hepatocyte damage (indicated by apoptosis, ballooning, cell cycle arrest) and with the stage of fibrosis. Elevated AST/ALT ratio is also associated with fibrosis. Therefore, it is not surprising that portal fibrosis defines a subgroup of NAFLD patients, who have higher risk for progressive liver disease and liver-related mortality [49]. Whether ductular reaction directly drives portal fibrosis as well as liver regeneration is still debated. In an experimental *in vivo* fibrogenesis model, ductular reaction was accompanied by collagen deposition, and the inhibition of progenitor cell expansion by TWEAK ameliorated the fibrogenic response [50].

NAFLD-RELATED CIRRHOSIS

There is clear evidence that a subgroup of NAFLD patients has progressive liver disease, which can lead to complete cirrhotic reconstruction of the liver, only patients with NASH may have such unfavorable outcome [51]. Now it is considered that a large portion of cryptogenic cirrhosis is actually burned out NASH [19]. Type II diabetes, obesity and other features of metabolic syndrome, such as dyslipidemia, higher BMI index, insulin resistance are more common in cryptogenic cirrhosis patients than in control group of HBV or HCV infection-related cirrhotic patients [52]; in a Mexican study, metabolic syndrome was six-fold more common in cryptogenic cirrhosis patients than in the control group [53]. In another large study, the overwhelming majority of liver biopsy samples from cryptogenic cirrhotic livers showed one or two histological features of NASH. Patients with NASH on average are 10 years younger than people with cryptogenic cirrhosis. Furthermore, high post-transplant recurrence of NASH has been observed in patients who underwent liver transplantation for cryptogenic cirrhosis [54]. Risk factors for recurrence were obesity and type II diabetes. All of these facts support that NASH-related fibrosis can insidiously evolve into complete cirrhosis with well-known complications, including the development of hepatocellular carcinoma (HCC) [55].

NAFLD AND HEPATOCELLULAR CARCINOMA

The first reports about the carcinogenic potential of NAFLD were published in the nineties of the previous century. The incidence of HCC is increasing continuously in the Western world. This raise has been attributed mostly to the increasing prevalence of HCV infection. However, due to the present achievements of antiviral therapies and more efficient control of spreading of viral infections, NAFLD may become the most important etiological factor of liver cancer. In fact, a recent study from Germany concluded that NAFLD has already surpassed chronic viral hepatitis as etiological factor [56]. These observations are strongly supported by large-scale epidemiological studies. According to an American investigation, men with a BMI of $35kg/m^2$ and above have 4.5 times higher risk of dying from HCC than people with average BMI [57]. Another meta-analysis described the relative risk of liver cancer to be 117% for overweight and 189% for obese patients [58]. Independent studies also emphasize the important role of diabetes mellitus in the development and progression of HCC; the risk of HCC was found 2-3 times higher in diabetic patients. Furthermore, diabetes has been described to act synergistically with other risk factors of HCC, namely viral hepatitis and alcoholic liver disease [59]. It is especially alarming that increased risk of HCC formation has been described in NAFLD patients without steatohepatitis and fibrosis, *i.e.* simple steatosis may be complicated with HCC [60]. Indirect evidences support the role of insulin resistance in hepato-carcinogenesis; the application of insulin-sensitizing chemicals may reduce the risk of HCC development or in later stage may improve the prognosis of patients with HCC. The finding that the prevalence of cirrhosis in NAFLD-related HCC is lower than that in ALD or HCV-related HCC suggests that HCC develops at an earlier stage of the chronic liver damage - cirrhosis sequence. The accurate role of NAFLD in the development of HCC is probably underestimated, because NAFLD as a synergist can contribute to the fibro- and carcinogenic potential of other liver-damaging mechanisms (viral hepatitis, ALD), and recent observations support that NAFLD can predispose patients to HCC in the absence of cirrhosis [59, 60]. Experimental models of NASH in rodents resulted in tumor formation without cirrhosis. There are also supporting data in humans showing that cirrhosis developed later in obese patients than in those with hepatitis C infection. Nevertheless, there was no difference in the occurrence of HCC between the two groups, indicating more efficient carcinogenic potential for NAFLD without cirrhosis. This raises serious concerns for the design of cancer-preventive screening of NAFLD patients.

There are some characteristic pathological features of HCC-s developing on the basis of NAFLD. The patients are usually older; the tumors are larger and better differentiated than HCCs induced by other etiologies. Interestingly, the WNT signaling pathway deregulation is quite rare. It has also been described that HCCs in non-cirrhotic livers are often developed in hepatocellular adenomas mostly in telangiectatic type [59]. This result suggests that HCCs in non-cirrhotic livers or at least a subgroup of them has a unique, distinct pathogenesis. Another group defined a distinctive histological variant of HCC, labeled with the name of steatohepatic hepatocellular carcinoma (SH-HCC) [61] (Fig. **9**). This type of tumor is characterized with histological features including macrovesicular steatosis, ballooning, Mallory-Denk bodies, and pericellular fibrosis, which are often present in NASH.

Although individually all of these lesions have been observed in "common" hepatocellular carcinomas, such combination was more common in NASH-related tumors. This relationship raises the possibility of a NASH - SH HCC histopathologic pathway, and the role of genomic imprinting or metabolic modification of the neoplastic pathway has been hypothesized. Insulin resistance and related factors can affect multiple growth and transcription factors.

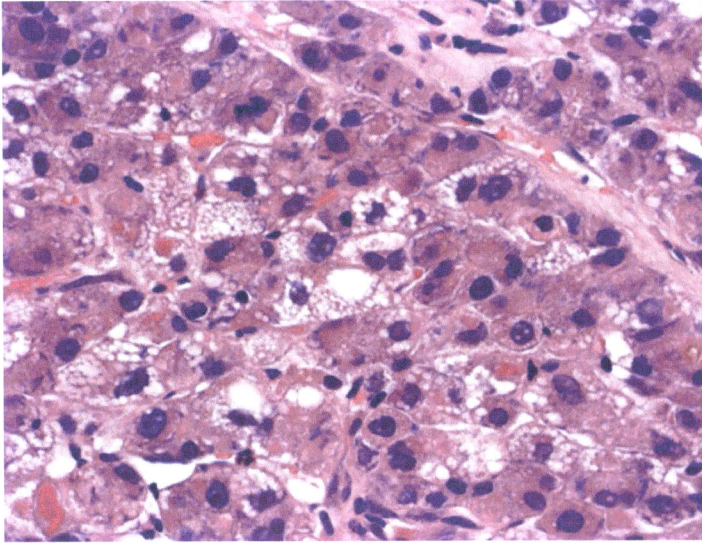

Fig. (9). Steatohepatic hepatocellular carcinoma. Well differentiated HCC with fat vacuoles and Mallory Denk bodies in the cytoplasm of the tumor cells.

PEDIATRIC NAFLD

The ratio of obese children grows rapidly worldwide and pediatric NAFLD is increasing in line with obesity since increased body weight, like in adults, is an important risk factor for this disease. There are no exact data, but it is estimated that the prevalence of NAFLD is approaching 10% among American and Asian children [62]. It is more common in boys, suggesting some hormone dependence. Familial clustering is also frequently observed, supporting the genetic background. NAFLD in children is mostly asymptomatic but subjects may complain about inconsistent abdominal pain, malaise, and fatigue. Acanthosis nigricans occurs quite often in children with NASH, and hepatomegaly can be recognized by physical examination [63]. Increased serum level of transaminases can be often but not always detected. Similarly to adults, histological examination is the only reliable way of diagnosing NAFLD, to distinguish simple steatosis from NASH. However, there are important histological differences between adult and pediatric NAFLD [64] which should be kept in mind during pathological evaluation of the liver biopsy (Table **2**).

Table 2. Major histological differences between adult and pediatric NASH.

	Adult	**Pediatric**
Steatosis	pericentral	Panacinar/azonal
Portal fibrosis	rare	common
Perisinusoidal fibrosis	common	rare

(Table 2) contd.....

	Adult	**Pediatric**
Inflammation	pericentral	periportal
Ballooning	common	rare

The distinction of two different types of pediatric NASH is now generally accepted. Type 1 pediatric NASH is consistent with the adult form of the disease. It is characterized by pericentral steatosis, perisinusoidal fibrosis, ballooning and the absence of portal lesions. This is the less common type of NASH in children. On the other hand, type 2 pediatric NASH, which is more often, is dominated by portal inflammation and fibrosis. Steatosis is present in the hepatocytes, but ballooning degeneration and perisinusoidal fibrosis are missing. This form of NASH is a more progressive disease which can lead eventually to complete cirrhosis. Off course, there are some overlapping forms of pediatric NASH, and in certain studies this is the most common form. There is general agreement that steatosis and portal inflammation are more severe in children compared to adults, but intralobular inflammation, ballooning is less common and milder. Ductular reaction is also present in pediatric NASH. Its extent and the number of intermediate hepatobiliary cells correlates with hepatocyte apoptosis and cell cycle arrest (p21 expression), suggesting that the activation of the hepatic progenitor cell compartment and its hepatocytic differentiation depend on the combination of hepatocyte injury and impaired regeneration [47]. Type 1 and 2 forms of NASH may have different pathogenesis, outcome and response to treatment. It is not known whether type 2 NASH changes to type 1 or adult form as the child ages. The distinct histological alterations between pediatric type 2 and adult form or pediatric type 1 NASH may reflect different etiology. In fact, obese adult male patients may have pediatric type NASH and this type 2 form of pediatric NASH is more prevalent among severely obese boys. That is obesity and male hormones might have some role in the etiology of this form of NASH. Interestingly, sucrose- and fructose-rich diet in rats induced mostly periportal damage [64]. This result suggests that inappropriate carbohydrate consumption, excessive drinking of sugar-rich beverages might play a role in the pathogenesis of pediatric form of NASH.

Steatosis is usually more severe in pediatric NASH. The extent of steatosis correlates with increasing portal inflammation, but it is not linked to any other histological parameters such as lobular inflammation, ballooning or fibrosis [65]. The failure of correlation between the extent of steatosis and progressive fibrosis is similar to the adult situation. The distribution of steatosis is also different in pediatric and adult form of NASH. While in adults fatty change affects mostly the pericentral hepatocytes, in children it is mostly panacinar or scattered, azonal. Surprisingly, azonal steatosis in children is associated with extensive ballooning and more common Mallory-Denk body formation, reflecting hepatocellular injury. It is important to emphasize that the extent of fibrosis, the progression of the disease in pediatric NAFLD is independent of the extent of steatosis [65], which can be quantitated by noninvasive techniques. Therefore, these imaging methods cannot replace histological examinations.

HISTOLOGICAL SCORING OF NAFLD

Recently histological examination of liver biopsy has been the golden standard for the diagnosis of NAFLD. Since scoring systems have been developed in most of the chronic liver diseases and used widely in everyday clinical practice, it is not surprising that classification systems correlating histology of NAFLD with disease outcome, response to therapy have been designed (Table **3**).

Table 3. Histological scoring of NAFLD.

	Major features	**Reference**
Matteoni's	simple, does not asses grading	Gastroenterology 116,1413,1999
Brunt's	grading, staging; does not cover entire spectrum of NAFLD	Am J. Gatroenterol 94,2467,1999
NAS	grading, staging; wide gray zone between steatosis and NASH, can not handle burned out NASH	Hepatology 41,1313,2005
SAF	steatosis, grading, staging; not applied to pediatric cases	Hepatology 56,1751,2012
PNHS	grading, no staging; designed for pediatric cases	J Hepatol 57,1312,2012

The first scoring system has been proposed by Matteoni *et al.* [66]. They distinguished four types of NAFLD including type 1: simple steatosis; type 2: steatosis and lobular inflammation; type 3: steatosis and hepatocellular ballooning; and type 4: steatosis with ballooning and either MDBs or fibrosis. This classification has not assessed disease severity or activity.

Later, Brunt *et al.* [67] designed a scoring system which distinguished, paralleling the concepts and terminology used for the classification of viral hepatitis, disease activity or grade based on the major histopathological lesions. The evaluated features are: steatosis, ballooning and inflammation, and a 5 tier (0-4) staging system based on the characteristic pattern of fibrosis.

This system could be applied only for the classification of NASH and did not cover the entire spectrum of NAFLD. These systems were not designed for the evaluation of pediatric liver samples, which may show different histological features. The recently most widely used NASH CRN system is mostly based on Brunt's scoring. It was designed by the National Institute of Diabetes & Digestive & Kidney Diseases (NIDDK) sponsored NASH Clinical Research Network (CRN) [33]. One of the major purposes of this project was to develop and validate a system of histological evaluation for the entire spectrum of NAFLD which could be applied to adult and pediatric samples and could be used for the assessment of therapy efficacy. The NASH CRN scoring system is based on the examination of 14 histological features, 4 of which were evaluated semi-quantitatively: steatosis (0-3), lobular inflammation (0-2), hepatocellular ballooning (0-2), and fibrosis (0-4).Other nine features were recorded as present or absent: microvesicular steatosis, microgranulomas, large lipogranulomas, portal inflammation, acidophil bodies, pigmented macrophages, megamitochondria, Mallory-Denk bodies, and glycogenated nuclei. The proposed NAFLD activity score (NAS) is the unweighted sum of steatosis, lobular inflammation and hepatocellular ballooning scores. The NAS score ≥ 5 correlated with a diagnosis of NASH, while the NAS scores < 3 were diagnosed as not NASH. This system is mostly used for comparative analysis of pretreatment and posttreatment biopsies of patients in therapeutic trials. It should not be used as an absolute severity scale and it was not intended to replace the pathologist's morphological diagnosis. NAS is not able of diagnosing NASH in patients with burned-out NASH in whom steatosis and inflammation is decreasing due to treatment and only fibrosis remained. Furthermore, there are major discrepancies in reports of the prevalence of NASH in obese subjects, ranging from 24% to 98%. The most likely explanation is the variable definition applied by pathologists. The most important task of the histological examination in case of NAFLD is the distinction between simple steatosis and NASH. Although the likelihood of NASH increases with NAS, there is a wide gray zone NAS 3-4. These failures encouraged Pierre Bedossa and colleagues [68] to propose another scoring system, which was named SAF (steatosis, activity and fibrosis). Since NAFLD is defined by fatty change, the presence of steatosis is the criterion (score 0-3) to enter into the algorithm. It is weighted by the grade of ballooning (0-2) and the extent of lobular inflammation (0-2). All patients with at least grade 1 steatosis were diagnosed to have NAFLD regardless of the grade of other criteria. The activity score (ballooning + lobular inflammation) made possible the discrimination of NASH, since all patients with NASH had A>2, while no patients with A<2 had NASH. There is no significant difference in the serum level of transaminases (ALT and AST) between individuals with normal liver and pure steatosis. This is why steatosis is not included into the activity score. The applied A score which is based on ballooning and lobular inflammation closely correlates with the level of transaminases. In the validation phase, the interobserver agreement for NASH was excellent by applying this activity scoring. The staging of fibrosis is practically the same as in NASH-CRN system, stage 0 - stage 4. The authors recommend that the SAF score dissociates the grade of steatosis, grade of activity and grade of fibrosis and this is more relevant than the simple distinction between NASH and non-NASH. It might be very useful to follow patients during clinical trials. So far this system has not been applied to pediatric NAFLD.

Originally the NAS score was designed to be used on pediatric cases as well. However, when NAS is applied to pediatric population, usually about half of the patients can only be categorized clearly, while the other half falls into borderline zone. This is not so surprising, since pediatric NAFLD is usually characterized by distinct histological features as compared to the adult type. Most importantly, portal inflammation may indicate a more severe disease in children. There are some other histological features *e.g.* hepatocyte ballooning that confer a more increased risk of disease progression than in adults, therefore it should carry more weight when developing a histological score. These considerations led Alkhouri *et al.* [69] to propose another scoring system designed especially for pediatric cases, called Pediatric NAFLD Histological Score (PNHS). PNHS score can be calculated by using the weighted sum of steatosis (1-3), ballooning (0-2), lobular inflammation (0-3) and portal inflammation (0-2). The score can be calculated by entering the individual histological features into the following website: http://rcc.simpal.com/RCEval.cgi?RCID=RPCxtv#Result. The PNHS value is prominently higher in the NASH group compared to the not NASH group and can be used for histological grading of pediatric NAFLD samples.

DIFFERENTIAL DIAGNOSTIC CONSIDERATIONS

The most common diagnostic problem is the differentiation between NASH and alcoholic hepatitis. The distinction in daily histopathological practice should not be made on pure morphological criteria. The diagnosis has to rely on clinicopathological data, but there are subtle histological differences which may be helpful to distinguish the two similar histological reactions [70]. Neutrophil granulocyte clusters, as component of the lobular inflammation, are much more common in alcoholic hepatitis as well as satellitosis, when polymorphonuclears are gathered around ballooned hepatocytes with MDBs. Although fatty change is mostly present in alcoholic hepatitis, it is not a diagnostic requirement. NAFLD is usually characterized by more extensive steatosis and less severe inflammatory changes. The special form of diffuse microvesicular steatosis also called as alcoholic foamy degeneration does not occur in NASH. Canalicular cholestasis and ductular reaction with polymorphonuclears, a consequence of biliary obstruction, is relatively common in alcoholic hepatitis, but not in NASH. Thickening and perivenular fibrosis of central veins, sclerosing hyaline necrosis (obliteration of central veins and necrosis of pericentral hepatocytes) can be seen also in alcoholic hepatitis [71]. Another helpful morphological sign is the presence of nuclear vacuolation (suggesting insulin resistance) which is seen in the majority of NAFLD samples but it is relatively rare in alcoholic liver disease [72]. Glycogenated nuclei can be observed even in NAFLD-related cirrhosis when most of the other histological characteristics have disappeared. Immunohistochemistry can also provide help. Protein tyrosine phosphatase 1B (PTB1B) is upregulated in the cytoplasm of hepatocytes in NASH samples [73]. On the contrary, the membranous insulin receptor staining was reported to disappear from the hepatocytes in NASH but not in alcoholic hepatitis. In addition to alcoholic hepatitis, there are several other conditions which can result in similar morphological alterations: metabolic disease (Wilson disease, tyrosinemia), drug toxicity (amiodarone, tamoxifen, glucocorticoids) surgical procedures (biliopancreatic diversion, jejunoileal bypass), parenteral nutrition, malnutrition *etc*. The knowledge of the clinico-pathological correlations is absolutely necessary to distinguish these lesions from different forms of NASH.

Portal inflammation and fibrosis can occur in adult NAFLD but usually it is limited. In case of intense periportal inflammatory reaction, other chronic diseases, mostly HCV-related cirrhosis, should be considered. HCV often causes steatosis as well, however the fatty change is less intense and the distribution is random, contrary to dominant pericentral steatosis in NAFLD. Serological and viral examinations can resolve these problems easily. However, NAFLD is a very common disease and the coexistence of NAFLD with other chronic liver diseases is frequently observed [9]. Clinical and pathological consequences of comorbidities are the subject of ongoing studies. The presence of NASH in chronic hepatitis C patients is correlated with advanced fibrosis and is more common in patients infected with HCV genotype 3 [9].

CONFLICT OF INTEREST

The author confirms that author has no conflict of interest to declare for this publication.

ACKNOWLEDGEMENTS

Declared none.

REFERENCES

[1]   Dyson JK, Anstee QM, McPherson S. Non-alcoholic fatty liver disease: a practical approach to diagnosis and staging. Frontline Gastroenterol 2014; 5(3): 211-8.
[http://dx.doi.org/10.1136/flgastro-2013-100403] [PMID: 25018867]

[2]   Sugimoto K, Takei Y. Clinicopathological features of non-alcoholic fatty liver disease. Hepatol Res 2011; 41(10): 911-20.
[http://dx.doi.org/10.1111/j.1872-034X.2011.00867.x] [PMID: 21951869]

[3]   Angulo P. Nonalcoholic fatty liver disease. N Engl J Med 2002; 346(16): 1221-31.
[http://dx.doi.org/10.1056/NEJMra011775] [PMID: 11961152]

[4]   Mofrad P, Contos MJ, Haque M, *et al.* Clinical and histologic spectrum of nonalcoholic fatty liver disease associated with normal ALT values. Hepatology 2003; 37(6): 1286-92.
[http://dx.doi.org/10.1053/jhep.2003.50229] [PMID: 12774006]

[5]   Saadeh S, Younossi ZM, Remer EM, *et al.* The utility of radiological imaging in nonalcoholic fatty liver disease. Gastroenterology 2002; 123(3): 745-50.
[http://dx.doi.org/10.1053/gast.2002.35354] [PMID: 12198701]

[6]   McPherson S, Jonsson JR, Cowin GJ. Magnetic resonance imaging and spectroscopy accurately estimate the severity of steatosis provided the stage of fibrosis is considered. J Hepatol 2009; 51: 389-97.

[7]   Tiniakos DG. Nonalcoholic fatty liver disease/nonalcoholic steatohepatitis: histological diagnostic criteria and scoring systems. Eur J Gastroenterol Hepatol 2010; 22(6): 643-50.
[PMID: 19478676]

[8]   Brunt EM. Pathology of nonalcoholic fatty liver disease. Nat Rev Gastroenterol Hepatol 2010; 7(4): 195-203.
[http://dx.doi.org/10.1038/nrgastro.2010.21] [PMID: 20195271]

[9]   Brunt EM, Ramrakhiani S, Cordes BG, *et al.* Concurrence of histologic features of steatohepatitis with other forms of chronic liver disease. Mod Pathol 2003; 16(1): 49-56.
[http://dx.doi.org/10.1097/01.MP.0000042420.21088.C7] [PMID: 12527713]

[10] Harmon RC, Tiniakos DG, Argo CK. Inflammation in nonalcoholic steatohepatitis. Expert Rev Gastroenterol Hepatol 2011; 5(2): 189-200.
[http://dx.doi.org/10.1586/egh.11.21] [PMID: 21476914]

[11] Nalbantoglu IL, Brunt EM. Role of liver biopsy in nonalcoholic fatty liver disease. World J Gastroenterol 2014; 20(27): 9026-37.
[PMID: 25083076]

[12] Gadd VL, Skoien R, Powell EE, *et al.* The portal inflammatory infiltrate and ductular reaction in human nonalcoholic fatty liver disease. Hepatology 2014; 59(4): 1393-405.
[http://dx.doi.org/10.1002/hep.26937] [PMID: 24254368]

[13] Carpino G, Renzi A, Onori P, Gaudio E. Role of hepatic progenitor cells in nonalcoholic fatty liver disease development: cellular cross-talks and molecular networks. Int J Mol Sci 2013; 14(10): 20112-30.
[http://dx.doi.org/10.3390/ijms141020112] [PMID: 24113587]

[14] Caldwell SH, Chang CY, Nakamoto RK, Krugner-Higby L. Mitochondria in nonalcoholic fatty liver disease. Clin Liver Dis 2004; 8(3): 595-617, x.
[http://dx.doi.org/10.1016/j.cld.2004.04.009] [PMID: 15331066]

[15] Brown KE, Washington K, Brunt EM. 2006.

[16]   Skelly MM, James PD, Ryder SD. Findings on liver biopsy to investigate abnormal liver function tests in the absence of diagnostic serology. J Hepatol 2001; 35(2): 195-9.
[http://dx.doi.org/10.1016/S0168-8278(01)00094-0] [PMID: 11580141]

[17]   Pillai AA, Rinella ME. Non-alcoholic fatty liver disease: is bariatric surgery the answer? Clin Liver Dis 2009; 13(4): 689-710.
[http://dx.doi.org/10.1016/j.cld.2009.07.012] [PMID: 19818313]

[18]   Levene AP, Goldin RD. The epidemiology, pathogenesis and histopathology of fatty liver disease. Histopathology 2012; 61(2): 141-52.
[http://dx.doi.org/10.1111/j.1365-2559.2011.04145.x] [PMID: 22372457]

[19]   Caldwell SH, Lee VD, Kleiner DE, *et al.* NASH and cryptogenic cirrhosis: a histological analysis. Ann Hepatol 2009; 8(4): 346-52.
[PMID: 20009134]

[20]   Schwimmer JB, Pardee PE, Lavine JE, Blumkin AK, Cook S. Cardiovascular risk factors and the metabolic syndrome in pediatric nonalcoholic fatty liver disease. Circulation 2008; 118(3): 277-83.
[http://dx.doi.org/10.1161/CIRCULATIONAHA.107.739920] [PMID: 18591439]

[21]   Chalasani N, Younossi Z, Lavine JE, *et al.* The diagnosis and management of non-alcoholic fatty liver disease: practice guideline by the American Gastroenterological Association, American Association for the Study of Liver Diseases, and American College of Gastroenterology. Gastroenterology 2012; 142(7): 1592-609.
[http://dx.doi.org/10.1053/j.gastro.2012.04.001] [PMID: 22656328]

[22]   Ratziu V, Bellentani S, Cortez-Pinto H, Day C, Marchesini G. A position statement on NAFLD/NASH based on the EASL 2009 special conference. J Hepatol 2010; 53(2): 372-84.
[http://dx.doi.org/10.1016/j.jhep.2010.04.008] [PMID: 20494470]

[23]   Gaidos JK, Hillner BE, Sanyal AJ. A decision analysis study of the value of a liver biopsy in nonalcoholic steatohepatitis. Liver Int 2008; 28(5): 650-8.
[http://dx.doi.org/10.1111/j.1478-3231.2008.01693.x] [PMID: 18331241]

[24]   Day CP, James OF. Steatohepatitis: a tale of two hits? Gastroenterology 1998; 114(4): 842-5.
[http://dx.doi.org/10.1016/S0016-5085(98)70599-2] [PMID: 9547102]

[25]   Neuschwander-Tetri BA. Hepatic lipotoxicity and the pathogenesis of nonalcoholic steatohepatitis: the central role of nontriglyceride fatty acid metabolites. Hepatology 2010; 52(2): 774-88.
[http://dx.doi.org/10.1002/hep.23719] [PMID: 20683968]

[26]   Argo CK, Al-Osaimi AM, Shah NL. Insulin resistance and deconditioning: further evidence of metabolic obesity in nonobese NASH. Hepatology 2010; 52 (Suppl. 1.): A630.

[27]   Puri P, Baillie RA, Wiest MM, *et al.* A lipidomic analysis of nonalcoholic fatty liver disease. Hepatology 2007; 46(4): 1081-90.
[http://dx.doi.org/10.1002/hep.21763] [PMID: 17654743]

[28]   Fujii H, Ikura Y, Arimoto J, *et al.* Expression of perilipin and adipophilin in nonalcoholic fatty liver disease; relevance to oxidative injury and hepatocyte ballooning. J Atheroscler Thromb 2009; 16(6): 893-901.
[http://dx.doi.org/10.5551/jat.2055] [PMID: 20032580]

[29]   Straub BK, Stoeffel P, Heid H, Zimbelmann R, Schirmacher P. Differential pattern of lipid droplet-associated proteins and de novo perilipin expression in hepatocyte steatogenesis. Hepatology 2008; 47(6): 1936-46.
[http://dx.doi.org/10.1002/hep.22268] [PMID: 18393390]

[30]   Tandra S, Yeh MM, Brunt EM, *et al.* Presence and significance of microvesicular steatosis in nonalcoholic fatty liver disease. J Hepatol 2011; 55(3): 654-9
[http://dx.doi.org/10.1016/j.jhep.2010.11.021] [PMID: 21172393]

[31]   Park JW, Jeong G, Kim SJ, Kim MK, Park SM. Predictors reflecting the pathological severity of non-alcoholic fatty liver disease: comprehensive study of clinical and immunohistochemical findings in younger Asian patients. J Gastroenterol Hepatol 2007; 22(4): 491-7.
[http://dx.doi.org/10.1111/j.1440-1746.2006.04758.x] [PMID: 17376039]

[32]   Wynn TA, Barron L. Macrophages: master regulators of inflammation and fibrosis. Semin Liver Dis 2010; 30(3): 245-57.
[http://dx.doi.org/10.1055/s-0030-1255354] [PMID: 20665377]

[33]   Brunt EM, Kleiner DE, Wilson LA, *et al.* Portal chronic inflammation in nonalcoholic fatty liver disease (NAFLD): a histologic marker of advanced NAFLD-Clinicopathologic correlations from the nonalcoholic steatohepatitis clinical research network. Hepatology 2009; 49(3): 809-20.
[http://dx.doi.org/10.1002/hep.22724] [PMID: 19142989]

[34]   Syn WK, Oo YH, Pereira TA, *et al.* Accumulation of natural killer T cells in progressive nonalcoholic fatty liver disease. Hepatology 2010; 51(6): 1998-2007.
[http://dx.doi.org/10.1002/hep.23599] [PMID: 20512988]

[35]   Richardson MM, Jonsson JR, Powell EE, *et al.* Progressive fibrosis in nonalcoholic steatohepatitis: association with altered regeneration and a ductular reaction. Gastroenterology 2007; 133(1): 80-90.
[http://dx.doi.org/10.1053/j.gastro.2007.05.012] [PMID: 17631134]

[36]   Yeh M, Brunt EM. Pathology of fatty liver disease: differential diagnosis of fatty liver disease. Diagn Histopathol 2008; 14: 586-97.
[http://dx.doi.org/10.1016/j.mpdhp.2008.09.005]

[37]   Machado MV, Cortez-Pinto H. Cell death and nonalcoholic steatohepatitis: where is ballooning relevant? Expert Rev Gastroenterol Hepatol 2011; 5(2): 213-22.
[http://dx.doi.org/10.1586/egh.11.16] [PMID: 21476916]

[38]   Feldstein AE, Canbay A, Angulo P, *et al.* Hepatocyte apoptosis and fas expression are prominent features of human nonalcoholic steatohepatitis. Gastroenterology 2003; 125(2): 437-43.
[http://dx.doi.org/10.1016/S0016-5085(03)00907-7] [PMID: 12891546]

[39]   Bechmann LP, Gieseler RK, Sowa JP, *et al.* Apoptosis is associated with CD36/fatty acid translocase upregulation in non-alcoholic steatohepatitis. Liver Int 2010; 30(6): 850-9.
[http://dx.doi.org/10.1111/j.1478-3231.2010.02248.x] [PMID: 20408954]

[40]   Oyadomari S, Harding HP, Zhang Y, Oyadomari M, Ron D. Dephosphorylation of translation initiation factor 2α enhances glucose tolerance and attenuates hepatosteatosis in mice. Cell Metab 2008; 7(6): 520-32.
[http://dx.doi.org/10.1016/j.cmet.2008.04.011] [PMID: 18522833]

[41]   Liu HY, Han J, Cao SY, *et al.* Hepatic autophagy is suppressed in the presence of insulin resistance and hyperinsulinemia: inhibition of FoxO1-dependent expression of key autophagy genes by insulin. J Biol Chem 2009; 284(45): 31484-92.
[http://dx.doi.org/10.1074/jbc.M109.033936] [PMID: 19758991]

[42]   Lackner C, Gogg-Kamerer M, Zatloukal K, Stumptner C, Brunt EM, Denk H. Ballooned hepatocytes in steatohepatitis: the value of keratin immunohistochemistry for diagnosis. J Hepatol 2008; 48(5): 821-8.
[http://dx.doi.org/10.1016/j.jhep.2008.01.026] [PMID: 18329127]

[43] Lackner C. Hepatocellular ballooning in nonalcoholic steatohepatitis: the pathologists perspective. Expert Rev Gastroenterol Hepatol 2011; 5(2): 223-31.
[http://dx.doi.org/10.1586/egh.11.8] [PMID: 21476917]

[44] Mallory FB. Cirrhosis of the liver. Five different types of lesions from which it may arise. Bull Johns Hopkins Hosp 1911; 22: 69-75.

[45] Zatloukal K, French SW, Stumptner C, *et al.* From Mallory to Mallory-Denk bodies: what, how and why? Exp Cell Res 2007; 313(10): 2033-49.
[http://dx.doi.org/10.1016/j.yexcr.2007.04.024] [PMID: 17531973]

[46] Neuschwander-Tetri BA. Hepatic lipotoxicity and the pathogenesis of nonalcoholic steatohepatitis: the central role of nontriglyceride fatty acid metabolites. Hepatology 2010; 52(2): 774-88.
[http://dx.doi.org/10.1002/hep.23719] [PMID: 20683968]

[47] Nobili V, Carpino G, Alisi A, *et al.* Hepatic progenitor cells activation, fibrosis, and adipokines production in pediatric nonalcoholic fatty liver disease. Hepatology 2012; 56(6): 2142-53.
[http://dx.doi.org/10.1002/hep.25742] [PMID: 22467277]

[48] Roskams TA, Theise ND, Balabaud C, *et al.* Nomenclature of the finer branches of the biliary tree: canals, ductules, and ductular reactions in human livers. Hepatology 2004; 39(6): 1739-45.
[http://dx.doi.org/10.1002/hep.20130] [PMID: 15185318]

[49] Gramlich T, Kleiner DE, McCullough AJ, Matteoni CA, Boparai N, Younossi ZM. Pathologic features associated with fibrosis in nonalcoholic fatty liver disease. Hum Pathol 2004; 35(2): 196-9.
[http://dx.doi.org/10.1016/j.humpath.2003.09.018] [PMID: 14991537]

[50] Jakubowski A, Ambrose C, Parr M, *et al.* TWEAK induces liver progenitor cell proliferation. J Clin Invest 2005; 115(9): 2330-40.
[http://dx.doi.org/10.1172/JCI23486] [PMID: 16110324]

[51] Farrell GC, Larter CZ. Nonalcoholic fatty liver disease: from steatosis to cirrhosis. Hepatology 2006; 43(2) (Suppl. 1): S99-S112.
[http://dx.doi.org/10.1002/hep.20973] [PMID: 16447287]

[52] Caldwell SH, Oelsner DH, Iezzoni JC, Hespenheide EE, Battle EH, Driscoll CJ. Cryptogenic cirrhosis: clinical characterization and risk factors for underlying disease. Hepatology 1999; 29(3): 664-9.
[http://dx.doi.org/10.1002/hep.510290347] [PMID: 10051466]

[53] Poonawala A, Nair SP, Thuluvath PJ. Prevalence of obesity and diabetes in patients with cryptogenic cirrhosis: a case-control study. Hepatology 2000; 32(4 Pt 1): 689-92.
[http://dx.doi.org/10.1053/jhep.2000.17894] [PMID: 11003611]

[54] Ong J, Younossi ZM, Reddy V, *et al.* Cryptogenic cirrhosis and posttransplantation nonalcoholic fatty liver disease. Liver Transpl 2001; 7(9): 797-801.
[http://dx.doi.org/10.1053/jlts.2001.24644] [PMID: 11552214]

[55] Baffy G, Brunt EM, Caldwell SH. Hepatocellular carcinoma in non-alcoholic fatty liver disease: an emerging menace. J Hepatol 2012; 56(6): 1384-91.
[http://dx.doi.org/10.1016/j.jhep.2011.10.027] [PMID: 22326465]

[56] Ertle J, Dechêne A, Sowa JP, *et al.* Non-alcoholic fatty liver disease progresses to hepatocellular carcinoma in the absence of apparent cirrhosis. Int J Cancer 2011; 128(10): 2436-43.
[http://dx.doi.org/10.1002/ijc.25797] [PMID: 21128245]

[57] Calle EE, Rodriguez C, Walker-Thurmond K, Thun MJ. Overweight, obesity, and mortality from cancer in a prospectively studied cohort of U.S. adults. N Engl J Med 2003; 348(17): 1625-38.
[http://dx.doi.org/10.1056/NEJMoa021423] [PMID: 12711737]

[58]　Larsson SC, Wolk A. Overweight, obesity and risk of liver cancer: a meta-analysis of cohort studies. Br J Cancer 2007; 97(7): 1005-8.
[PMID: 17700568]

[59]　Paradis V, Zalinski S, Chelbi E, *et al.* Hepatocellular carcinomas in patients with metabolic syndrome often develop without significant liver fibrosis: a pathological analysis. Hepatology 2009; 49(3): 851-9.
[http://dx.doi.org/10.1002/hep.22734] [PMID: 19115377]

[60]　Guzman G, Brunt EM, Petrovic LM, Chejfec G, Layden TJ, Cotler SJ. Does nonalcoholic fatty liver disease predispose patients to hepatocellular carcinoma in the absence of cirrhosis? Arch Pathol Lab Med 2008; 132(11): 1761-6.
[PMID: 18976012]

[61]　Salomao M, Yu WM, Brown RS Jr, Emond JC, Lefkowitch JH. Steatohepatitic hepatocellular carcinoma (SH-HCC): a distinctive histological variant of HCC in hepatitis C virus-related cirrhosis with associated NAFLD/NASH. Am J Surg Pathol 2010; 34(11): 1630-6.
[PMID: 20975341]

[62]　Schwimmer JB, Deutsch R, Kahen T, Lavine JE, Stanley C, Behling C. Prevalence of fatty liver in children and adolescents. Pediatrics 2006; 118(4): 1388-93.
[http://dx.doi.org/10.1542/peds.2006-1212] [PMID: 17015527]

[63]　Rashid M, Roberts EA. Nonalcoholic steatohepatitis in children. J Pediatr Gastroenterol Nutr 2000; 30(1): 48-53.
[http://dx.doi.org/10.1097/00005176-200001000-00017] [PMID: 10630439]

[64]　Takahashi Y, Fukusato T. Pediatric nonalcoholic fatty liver disease: overview with emphasis on histology. World J Gastroenterol 2010; 16(42): 5280-5.
[http://dx.doi.org/10.3748/wjg.v16.i42.5280] [PMID: 21072890]

[65]　Carter-Kent C, Brunt EM, Yerian LM, *et al.* Relations of steatosis type, grade, and zonality to histological features in pediatric nonalcoholic fatty liver disease. J Pediatr Gastroenterol Nutr 2011; 52(2): 190-7.
[http://dx.doi.org/10.1097/MPG.0b013e3181fb47d3] [PMID: 21240012]

[66]　Matteoni CA, Younossi ZM, Gramlich T, Boparai N, Liu YC, McCullough AJ. Nonalcoholic fatty liver disease: a spectrum of clinical and pathological severity. Gastroenterology 1999; 116(6): 1413-9.
[http://dx.doi.org/10.1016/S0016-5085(99)70506-8] [PMID: 10348825]

[67]　Brunt EM, Janney CG, Di Bisceglie AM, Neuschwander-Tetri BA, Bacon BR. Nonalcoholic steatohepatitis: a proposal for grading and staging the histological lesions. Am J Gastroenterol 1999; 94(9): 2467-74.
[http://dx.doi.org/10.1111/j.1572-0241.1999.01377.x] [PMID: 10484010]

[68]　Bedossa P, Poitou C, Veyrie N, *et al.* Histopathological algorithm and scoring system for evaluation of liver lesions in morbidly obese patients. Hepatology 2012; 56(5): 1751-9.
[http://dx.doi.org/10.1002/hep.25889] [PMID: 22707395]

[69]　Alkhouri N, De Vito R, Alisi A, *et al.* Development and validation of a new histological score for pediatric non-alcoholic fatty liver disease. J Hepatol 2012; 57(6): 1312-8.
[http://dx.doi.org/10.1016/j.jhep.2012.07.027] [PMID: 22871498]

[70]　Brunt EM, Tiniakos DG. Pathological features of NASH. Front Biosci 2005; 10: 1475-84.
[PMID: 15769638]

[71]　Yip WW, Burt AD. Alcoholic liver disease. Semin Diagn Pathol 2006; 23(3-4): 149-60.
[http://dx.doi.org/10.1053/j.semdp.2006.11.002] [PMID: 17355088]

[72]   Brunt EM, Tiniakos DG. Alcoholic and non-alcoholic fatty liver disease. In: Odze RD, Goldblum JR, Crawford JM, Eds. pathology of the GI tract, liver biliary tract and pancreas. Philadelphia: Saunders 2009; pp. 1087-114.
[http://dx.doi.org/10.1016/B978-141604059-0.50044-8]

[73]   Sanderson SO, Smyrk TC. The use of protein tyrosine phosphatase 1B and insulin receptor immunostains to differentiate nonalcoholic from alcoholic steatohepatitis in liver biopsy specimens. Am J Clin Pathol 2005; 123(4): 503-9.
[http://dx.doi.org/10.1309/1PX2LMPQUH1EE12U] [PMID: 15743753]

CHAPTER 5

Pathophysiology of NAFLD

Gabriella Par[*]

First Department of Medicine, University of Pécs, Pécs, Hungary

Abstract: *Non-alcoholic fatty liver disease* (NAFLD) and its more severe form, *non-alcoholic steatohepatitis* (NASH) are common causes of chronic liver disease and major components of the metabolic syndrome. NASH is characterized by the presence of steatosis with necro-inflammation and fibrosis, progressing to cirrhosis and hepatocellular carcinoma. The pathogenesis of NAFLD and NASH originally was regarded as "two-hit" model, suggesting that the accumulation of fat in the liver cells (steatosis) as the first sensitizes the liver to a second hit that triggers a cascade of tissue damages (necro-inflammation and fibrosis). Today, it is widely accepted, that a more complex process, involving multiple parallel metabolic hits is responsible for tissue injury, and that other factors promote disease progression. Thus, now, *lipotoxicity, mitochondrial dysfunction, insulin resistance and oxidative stress* are considered as the main mechanisms in the pathogenesis of NASH. Reactive oxygen species (ROS), lipid peroxidation products and cytokines are involved in the progression, including the migration of resident hepatic pro-fibrogenic cells, which leads to fibrosis. Hepatocyte death, inflammation, and cellular senescence also play a role in the pathogenesis of the disease. The interaction between inflammatory cells including Th17 cells and other cell types such as hepatocytes, stellate cells, hepatic progenitor cells and ductular components is of pivotal importance, as well as the reactivation of developmental morphogenic signaling pathway, the hedgehog.

Keywords: Non-alcoholic fatty liver disease, Non-alcoholic steatohepatitis, Pathogenesis.

INTRODUCTION

The pathogenesis of non-alcoholic fatty liver disease (NAFLD) and its more severe form, non-alcoholic steatohepatitis (NASH), was regarded originally as a "**two-hit**" model, suggesting that the accumulation of fat in the liver cells (steatosis) as the *first hit* sensitizes the liver to a *second hit* that triggers a cascade of tissue injuries (necro-inflammation and fibrosis) [1]. Today, it is

[*] **Corresponding author Gabriella Par:** First Department of Medicine, University of Pécs, Pécs, Hungary; Tel: +36 72 536 000; Fax: +36 72 536 148; E-mail: pargabriella@gmail.com

Tatjana Ábel & Gabriella Lengyel (Eds.)
All rights reserved-© 2017 Bentham Science Publishers

widely accepted, that a more complex process, involving multiple parallel metabolic hits is responsible for tissue injury, and that other factors promote disease progression [2 - 5] (Fig. **1**).

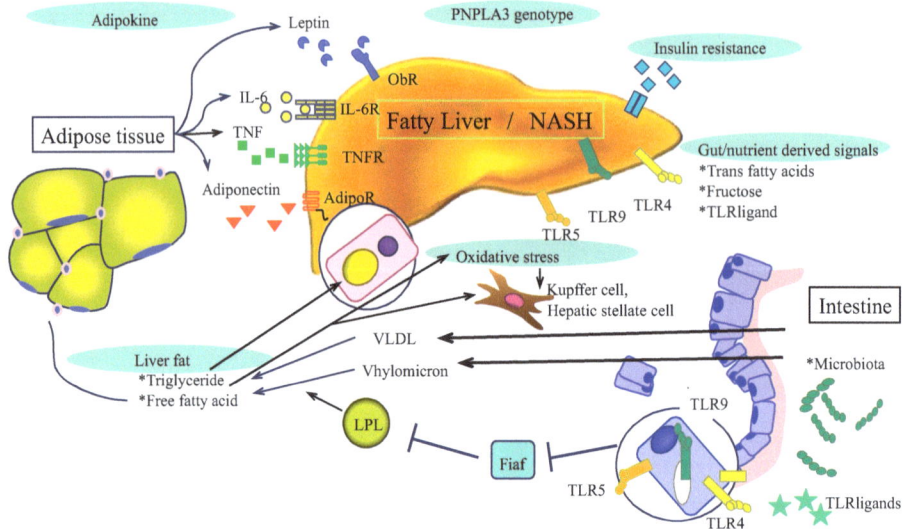

Fig. (1). Multiple parallel hit theory of NAFLD.

Genome-wide association studies have suggested the pivotal importance of patatin-like phospholipase 3 (PNPL3) gene polymorphism in NAFLD and the inflammation, that could even precede steatosis. Obesity and diabetes induce insulin resistance, adipocyte proliferation and changes in intestinal flora. Cytokines, such as IL-6 and TNF-α produced by adipocytes affect hepatocyte fat content and liver inflammatory environment. Gut derived signals are affected by ingested fatty acids, fructose, or TLR ligands. Free fatty acids and triglycerides induce ER stress and oxidative stress, resulting in inflammation and fibrogenesis in the liver.

Free fatty acids, cytokines, oxidative stress, apoptosis and gut-derived lipopolysaccharides (LPSs) trigger an *inflammatory response and liver damage* in NAFLD and NASH. *Reactive oxygen species* (ROS) generated during free fatty acid (FAA) metabolism in microsomes, peroxisomes and mitochondria are the source of oxidative stress. ROS, lipid peroxidation products and cytokines are involved in the progression of simple steatosis to NASH, *insulin resistance and mitochondrial dysfunction* which are of pivotal importance in the pathogenesis. In addition, ROS induce the migration of resident hepatic pro-fibrogenic cells, resulting in *fibrosis* [6 - 8].

EXTRAHEPATIC AND INTRAHEPATIC MECHANISMS IN NAFLD

According to Byrne *et al.'s* conception [9], ***extrahepatic and intrahepatic mechanisms*** contribute to the development of NAFLD and NASH. We first discuss these basic factors of the pathogenesis.

Extrahepatic Mechanisms

Regarding *the lipolysis and non-esterified ("free") fatty acids (FFAs),* it is generally accepted, that increased delivery of FFAs to the liver from peripheral (adipose) tissues is fundamental to the development of NAFLD. Approximately, 60% of fat deposited in hepatocytes is generated from adipose tissue sources. In subjects with **insulin resistance** (IR), there is a *failure of insulin mediated suppression of hormone-sensitive lipase (HSL) resulting in uncontrolled lipolysis in the adipose tissue and increased FFA delivery to the liver* [10].

Saturated fatty acids (SFAs) are capable of exacerbating IR at the insulin receptor level, due to translocation of the protein kinase C delta isoform (PKCdelta) from the cytosol to the membrane compartment leading to impaired insulin receptor substrate (IRS) / PI3K (phosphoinositide 3-kinase) activation. High dietary saturated fatty acids are associated with IR, NAFLD and cardiovascular (CV) risk [11].

*Polyunsaturated fatty acids (**n-3 PUFAs**)* in the diet have a protective role in the pathogenesis of NAFLD and may be a potential therapeutic target [9].

Sterol-regulatory-element binding protein 1c (**SREPB-1c**) is a transcription factor for *de novo* lipogenesis and is negatively regulated by **n-3 PUFAs**, thus the activities of key enzymes for FAA synthesis are down-regulated with decreased hepatic fat deposition. In addition, n-3 PUFAs negatively regulate the activity of a *glucose-responsive-transcription factor* (carbohydrate-responsive-elemet-binding protein, **ChREBP**), disrupting its translocation from the cytosol to the nucleus. High dietary intake of simple *sugars or fructose* increases *de novo* lipogenesis [12].

Phosphatidylcholine (**PC**) consists of medium-chain saturated fatty acids, and it is essential for the synthesis of VLDL particles and for the incorporation of neutral lipids into these particles. PC deficiency is associated with hepatic fat deposition secondary to the impaired export of VLDL particles [13].

Intrahepatic Mechanisms

There are several enzymes and transcription factors of *de novo* lipogenesis that represent the intrahepatic mechanisms for the development of NAFLD [9].

Enzymes

*Acetyl-CoA carboxylase **(ACC)** activity* is regulated by the cell energy status, insulin and the availability of NADPH. When cell energy is low with high AMP/ATP ratio, ACC is kept in its inactive phosphorylated form and acetyl–CoA is Channeled to β-oxidation and ketogenesis for energy production. ACC is under hormonal control by insulin. Insulin stimulates protein phosphatase 2A which dephosphorylates ACC, activating ACC and promoting lipogenesis. There are two isoforms of ACC: **ACC1** in the cytosol, is expressed in liver and adipose tissue, while **ACC2,** the mitochondrial isoform is expressed mainly in muscle and liver, and is involved in the negative regulation of mitochondrial β-oxidation. Fatty acid synthesis takes place in the cytosol, thus only ACC1 is important in the *de novo* pathway for fatty acid synthesis [14].

*Fatty acid synthase **(FAS)*** is the last key enzyme in *de novo* fatty acid synthesis [15].

*Stearoyl-CoA desaturase-1 **(SCD-1)**:* The synthesis of mono-unsaturated fatty acids (components of triglycerides, cholesterol esters) is catalyzed by SCD-1 [9].

Diacylglycerol acyltransferase-2 **(DGAT-2)** catalyzes the final step in *triglyceride synthesis.* Interestingly, its inhibition in db/db mice on methionine choline deficient (MCD) diet resulted in worsening inflammation, hepatocyte injury and fibrosis. Now, it has become accepted, that triglyceride itself may not be harmful, instead it protects the liver from lipid toxicity and toxic free-radicals by buffering hepatic fatty acids into the synthesis of triglycerides [16].

Transcription Factors

Sterol-regulatory-element binding protein 1c **(SREBP-1c)** is a positive transcription factor for ACC and FAS genes and its abnormality plays a pathogenetic role in NAFLD. Its overexpression in adult rats causes an increase in FAA synthesis and fat deposition, and it also stimulates gene expression for fatty acid elongation and triglyceride synthesis. The effect of insulin on lipogenesis is mediated *via* SREBP-1c activity [17].

Insulin induced gene-1(INSIG-1) is expressed in hepatocytes and adipocytes and inhibits lipogenesis and limits triglyceride deposition in hepatocytes. The benefits of peroxisome-proliferator-activated receptor-gamma (PPAR-γ) agonists in NASH may be due to the regulation of INSIG-1 [9, 18].

SH2-containing inositol phosphatase-2(SHIP-2) is an insulin-signal-regulatory phosphatase [19].

Phosphatase and tensin homolog deleted on chromosome 10 (**PTEN**) is a tumor-suppressor protein with phosphatase activity, and exerts a regulatory effect on the insulin signaling pathways. The physiological function of PTEN is to dephosphorylate the second messengers, thereby downregulating or terminating insulin signaling of PI3K. Overexpression of PTEN exerts inhibitory effects on insulin signaling [20]. In contrast, down-regulation of PTEN increases glucose uptake in fat and muscle in response to insulin [21]. The lack of PTEN activity, the increased hepatocyte fatty acid uptake, fatty acid synthesis and esterification of fatty acids to triglyceride may lead to excessive fat deposition in the liver [22].

Unsaturated non-esterified free fatty acids (FAAs) decrease the expression of PTEN *via* the activation of *mammalian target of rapamycin* (**mTOR**) and/or **NF-kB** pathways [23].

mTOR when activated down-regulates insulin signaling in insulin responsive tissue [24]. As insulin activates the mTOR, it seems that upregulation of this pathway may be due to the increased fasting insulin level associated with high dietary fat and insulin resistance. Increased FFA delivery upregulates the mTOR pathway, thus exacerbates IR [25].

Carbohydrate-responsive-element-binding protein (**ChREBp**) is a glucose-responsive transcription factor, which is controlled by glucose and regulates the translocation of L-pyruvate kinase from cytosol to the nucleus [26].

Liver X receptor-α (**LXR-α**) is a member of the nuclear receptor family that plays an important role in lipogenesis, it exerts transcriptional control on SREBP-1c and indirectly on ACC and FAS [27].

GENETICS AND EPIGENETIC EFFECTS

Genetics

Genom-wide association studies (GWAS) have confirmed the importance of *patatin-like phospholipase 3 (PNPLA3) gene* polymorphisms in NAFLD [28].

This polymorphism differentiates between simple steatosis and NASH. Patients with the single nucleotide polymorphism (SNP) rs738409 G/G genotype may progress not only to steatosis but to NASH. The function of PNPLA3 is not well known, but it may be that PNPLA3 acts as a downstream target gene of sterol-regulated binding protein 1c (SREBP-1c) to mediate the stimulation of lipid accumulation [29, 30].

Epigenetic Effects

Burdge *et al.* [31, 32] showed for the first time that modification of intrauterin nutrition during gestation affects *epigenetic regulation* of metabolic genes and has the potential to modify the disesase phenotype. Their findings revealed that intrauterine nutrition may modify hepatic lipogenesis as prenatal nutrition induces differential changes to the methylation of individual CpG dinucleotides in the hepatic PPAR-γ promoter, altering mRNA levels of the PPAR-α gene. The high fat diet in the pregnant mother may result in increased placental transfer of fatty acids to the fetus, enhancing hepatic lipogenesis and oxidative stress in the vulnerable fetal liver. This process may increase the demand for *methyl donors* to promote cell growth, and if those are not available, epigenetic changes in gene expression may result in a disposition to NAFLD in the developing offspring.

The mitochondrial genome is susceptible to oxidative damage due to the absence of protective histones and incomplete repair mechanisms. Mitochondrial dysfunction caused by changes in mDNA or altered expression of nuclear genes could cause increase in oxidative stress which may alter nuclear gene expression and cell function. Thus, the early nutrition may influence the flux of fatty acids to the developing fetal liver and increases susceptibility of the liver to NAFLD induced by a second post-natal exposure to a high-fat diet. Taken together, evidence from both epidemiological and experimental animal studies demonstrates that metabolic syndrome onset is increasingly likely following exposure to suboptimal nutrition during critical periods of development, as observed in maternal obesity. Thus, the developmental priming of the metabolic syndrome provides a common origin for this multifactorial disorder [33].

ADIPOKINES

Adipokines are multifunctional cytokines primarily derived from adipose tissue, that can be considered a complex organ, involving in the control of metabolic, immunologic and inflammatory responses.

Adiponectin is produced in white adipose tissue and its expression and secretion increase during adipocyte differentiation. It decreases *de novo* fatty acid synthesis, but increases β-oxidation and decreases triglyceride synthesis, and exerts a direct anti-inflammatory effect by decreasing TNF-α production. NAFLD patients have decreased expression of adiponectin receptors in the liver and lower serum adiponectin level as compared with simple steatosis [34, 35]. Adiponectin levels inversely correlate with visceral obesity and IR, and weight loss is an inducer of adiponectin synthesis. Pro-inflammatory cytokines TNF-α and IL6 suppress adiponectin, which has anti-inflammmatory and anti-diabetic properties. Serum adiponectin levels were found to be low in NAFLD and much lower in NASH patients [36].

Leptin is another adipokine; its levels correlate with body fat mass and adipocyte size [37]. Leptin production is regulated by food intake, insulin and sex hormones. Insulin increases its secretion similarly as ovarian sex steroids and proinflammmatory cytokines (TNF-α, IL-1), while testosterone inhibits leptin production. Leptin acts on hypothalamic cells, inhibits anabolic and activates catabolic pathways, inhibits appetite, increases basal metabolism, regulates pancreatic cell function and insulin secretion, and affects differentiation of T helper 1 cells in lymph nodes. As adiponectin and leptin have antagonistic effects on inflammation and fibrogenesis, their ratio may distinguish NASH from NAFLD [38].

OXIDATIVE AND ENDOPLASMIC RETICULUM STRESS

The increased flux of *free fatty acids* (FFAs) in hepatocytes represents the basic mechanism in hepatocyte dysfunction leading to progression in NASH. The excess FFA traffic is a consequences of increased dietary intake of saturated fatty acids and *de novo* lipogenesis and adipose lipolysis due to insulin resistance and impairment of compensatory oxidative processes [39]. The result is the generation of *toxic lipid metabolites,* such as *The result is the generation of toxic lipid metabolites, such as diacylglycerol ceramides and oxidized cholesterol metabolites which act as reactive oxygen species , ceramides and oxidized cholesterol metabolites* which act as *reactive oxygen species* (ROS). Mitochondrial, peroxisomal and microsomal origin **ROS** in NASH induce *oxidative stress,* that results in apoptosis and damage of nuclear and mitochondrial DNA.

Although its role in NASH is not fully understood [40], levels of **iron** are elevated in NASH, which is an inducer of oxidative stress. George *et al.* first showed that HFE gene mutations were associated with **increased hepatic iron**, acinar inflammation and steatosis in NASH [41]. Later contradictory results appeared in this field, yet recent studies have shown that increased hepatic iron in NASH is associated with IR and liver diseases most commonly associated with IR are also associated with iron overload. A correlation was found between serum ferritin levels and the presence of NASH and an association was found between ferritin and iron overload [42 - 44]. However, as ferritin is an acute phase protein, it may be a marker of the obesity-related pro-inflammatory state rather than iron overload in NASH [45].

Elevated plasma **citrate** levels in NAFLD promote iron mediated *hydroxyl radical* formation *in vitro* [46]. Excess fatty acids result in the elevation of pyruvate and acetyl-CoA that increases the formation of citrate, which induces iron related oxidative stress.

Mitochondrial fatty acid oxidation is not inhibited until respiration is severely impaired resulting in accelerated ROS production, until mitochondria are lost. Thus, *mitochondria are the main source of oxidative stress.* ER stress can induce superoxide and hydrogen peroxide with cytochrome P450, and peroxisomes can induce cytosolic hydrogen peroxide associated with fatty acid oxidation. The production of large amounts of ROS in the inner membrane of mitochondria can attack proximal *mitochondrial DNA,* causing mutations and finally apoptosis. Decreases in mitochondrial DNA and DNA-encoded peptides are characteristic findings in NASH, while the mitochondrial DNA content is increased in simple fatty liver. The complementary activation of mitochondrial DNA in fatty liver might help to protect the liver from inflammation, whereas a decrease in NASH induces progressive inflammation and fibrosis [4, 47].

The cytotoxic ROS and lipid peroxidation products can diffuse into the extracellular space affecting Kupffer cells and HSCs, and induce activation of NFκB which induces the synthesis of TNF-α, IL-1r, and IL-8. Kupffer cells in NASH patients produce TGF-β resulting in a fibrogenic myofibroblast-like phenotype. HSC activation is associated with the loss of cytoplasmic lipid droplets, (retinyl esters and triglycerides). Autophagy is upregulated in activated HSCs as an adaptive response to cellular stress to generate intracellular nutrients and energy [48, 49].

INSULIN RESISTANCE (IR)

IR is a central mechanism and several genetic and environmental factors interact to the development of IR. In NAFLD, obesity-related adipocyte dysfunction occurs with increased calorie intake and adipocyte hypertrophy and altered levels of adipokines [5, 50, 51]. IR results in increased lipolysis in adipose tissue, increased FFA uptake by hepatocytes and increased triglyceride synthesis. Mitochondrial fat oxidation and export of VLDL particles are not able to match triglyceride synthesis, resulting in a net fat deposition in the hepatocyte. The increased fatty acid oxidation in the mitochondria and peroxisome results in the generation of toxic oxygen free radicals, severe mitochondrial dysfunction with structural abnormalities, and ATP depletion. TNF-α induces IR by means of serine phosphorylation of IRS-1 (insulin receptor substrate-1), which exerts an inhibitory effect on the downstream propagation of insulin signals [52]. Another mechanism for TNF-α-induced IR is through the activation of the IKK-β pathway. The activation of this pathway results in downstream NFκ-B activation with inflammation and IR. Endoplasmic reticulum (ER) is a cellular organelle for the synthesis, storage and transport of proteins. ER stress directly activates the IKK/NFκB pathways *via* interactions with IRE-1, thus it induces inflammation and IR [53]. The increased hepatocyte *triglyceride formation* which occurs in parallel with the generation of toxic metabolites is now regarded as a protective mechanism to counter lipotoxicity [4, 5].

OBESITY

Obesity induces endoplasmic stress (ER), which leads to a compensatory response causes hyperactivation of c-jun terminal kinase (JNK) and further impairment of insulin signaling. Hyperinsulinemia decreases insulin signaling, which promotes steatosis. Insulin resistant adipose tissue produces excessive amounts of FFA *via* lipolysis creating lipotoxic metabolites. FFAs activate TLR4, and destabilize lysosomal membranes, causing cathepsin B release and leading to apoptosis. At the same time, peripheral adipose tissue produces damaging pro-inflammatory cytokines (TNF-α, IL-6), which results in chronic inflammation and IR [54].

Recently, Peverill *et al.* [5] reported a comprehensive review on the evolving concepts of NASH, focusing on lipotoxicity, IR, oxidative stress, hepatocyte death, inflammation, fibrosis, and cellular senescence. The authors emphasized that both the apoptosis and the interaction between immune cells and hepatocytes, stellate cells (HSCs), hepatic progenitor cells (HPCs) and ductular components are of basic importance in NASH pathogenesis.

APOPTOSIS

Apoptosis is a programmed form of cell death with minimal leakage of cellular components into the extra-cellular space, and is associated with low level of inflammatory response [55, 56]. Lipotoxicity leads to cell injury and death *via* apoptosis or necrosis and that is an important stimulus for inflammation and fibrosis in NASH. Cell death is manifested as hepatocyte ballooning and the appearance of apoptotic bodies and spotty necrosis. Necrosis is characterized by cellular swelling and release of cellular components, following disruption of organelles and surface membrane integrity. Although necrosis is a potent pro-inflammatory factor, apoptosis represents the major mechanism of cell death in NASH. Increased levels of apoptosis can be seen in obese patients with NASH as compared with controls. Apoptosis levels correlate with serum FAA levels, FFAs sensitize hepatocytes to the cytotoxic effects of death ligands (TNF-related apoptosis inducing ligand, TRAIL). The expression of the death receptor Fas (CD95) was higher in NASH than in simple steatosis [57 - 59]. Higher circulating FAA levels were associated with higher Fas expression. FAAs promote mitochondrial dysfunction through the ROS production and JNK activation exacerbates ROS accumulation, which induces hepatocyte apoptosis [60]. FAAs activate the lysosomal pathway increasing permeability and cathepsin B release. It has been shown that saturated FFAs induce increased ER stress response seen in NASH, and leads to apoptosis through release of Ca^2 from ER, ROS production, induction of pro-apoptotic transcription factors and increased JNK signaling [61].

Apoptosis is pro-fibrogenic; apoptotic bodies increase HSC activation *in vitro* and lead to the increased production of TGFβ, a potent profibrogenic cytokine [62].

(See later for the ballooning and the role of hedgehog activation in fibrogenesis)

HEPATOCYTE SENESCENCE

Senescence - a cellular stress response and an irreversible cell cycle arrest, that limit the proliferation of severely damaged cells - is also a mediator of disease progression in NASH [63, 64]. Oxidative stress can induce apoptosis, which is featured by the increased expression of cyclin-dependent kinase (CDK) inhibitors (**p21CI1, p16INK4a**) and formation of senescence-associated heterochromatin foci (**SAHF**) and DNA damage foci within the nucleus, and increased lysosomal beta-glactosidase activity. Accelerated telomere shortening as an inducer of senescence may occur in oxidative stress. Senescent cells mediate disease progression through the secretion of pro-inflammatory factors that affect the microenvironment, representing the adoption of a "senescence-associated secretory phenotype" (**SASP**) [65]. Senescent cells secrete proinflammmatory cytokines (IL-6, IL-8), matrix degrading enzymes (MMPs) and growth factors (HGF, PDGF, CTGF). Chemotactic factors that recruit inflammatory cells to the site of injury represent an important component of the SASP. These SASP products play a role in the progression of NASH. Hepatocyte **p21** expression and increased nuclear sizes were significantly associated with the stage of fibrosis in NAFLD biopsies [66]. It was also shown that areas of increased p21 expression correlated with increased αSMA expression, suggest a link between senescence and HSC activation, which leads to fibrosis. Senescence may have a role in limiting fibrosis and stimulating regeneration as well. In CCl_4 induced liver injury in mice, initial activation of HSCs was followed by the adoption of a senescent HSC phenotype with associated up-regulation of MMPs and down-regulation of ECM components, thus leading to reversion of fibrosis [67]. Finally, in NAFLD biopsies increased hepatic progenitor cell (HPC) expansion was found in association with increased stage of the disease. The degree of ductular reaction (DR) was associated with the extent of replicative arrest (p21 expression) [68].

IMMUNE RESPONSE

The inflammation in NASH involves both the innate and adaptive immune systems. The cascade begins with hepatocyte injury and lipotoxicity and propagated by cellular apoptosis and hepatocyte senescence, culminating in activation of HSCs and fibrosis. The **innate immune** response is mediated by neutrophils, macrophages (Kupffer cells), natural killer (NK) cells, and natural killer T (NKT) cells.

Macrophages directly activate hepatic stellate cells (HSCs) through the release of IL-6 and TGFβ. Furthermore, they promote HSC apoptosis (*via* TRAIL) and matrix degradation (*via* MMP-13 and MMP-9), and are considered as the source of proinflammmatory cytokines TNFα and IL-12. *Neutrophils* take part in the initial inflammatory response, mediated *via* the IL-1 receptor, while *NK cells* induce apoptosis of both HSC-s and hepatocytes *via* production of IFN-γ [69, 70]. *NKT cells* are activated by lipids, induce an adaptive immune response and may contribute to the development of fibrosis in NASH [71, 72].

In the **adaptive immune response,** *CD4⁺ T* cells may interact with fibroblasts and macrophages, while *CD8⁺ T cells* increase HSC activation by amplifying local cytokine milieu. *B cells* secrete profibrogenic cytokines IL-4, IL-6 IL-13. *HSC-s* express chemokines that recruit leukocytes, and facilitate interactions between leukocytes and fibroblasts [72]. *HSC*-s act as antigen presenting cells, stimulate T cells, and thus the inflammatory response and they cause a dysregulated tissue repair response that results in fibrosis. In portal infiltrates of NAFLD patients predominantly CD8⁺ Tcell, CD68⁺ macrophages, with smaller numbers of CD4⁺ T cells, CD20⁺ B cells and CD56⁺ NK cells have been demonstrated to support the role of the adaptive immune response in the disease [73, 74].

Toll-like Receptors

Since in NASH there is no recognized antigen or pathogen which evokes the immune response, the so-called "*sterile inflammation*" plays a role in the disease. Excess FFAs and oxidative stress, hepatocyte injury (apoptosis and/or necrosis) and hepatocyte senescence are the primary causes of the response, where the metabolic dysregulation is associated with obesity and IR promotes the chronic inflammatory state [5].

In "**steril inflammation**" the release of *damage associated molecular patterns* (DAMPs) from injured (necrotic or apoptotic) cells trigger the immune reaction. DAMPs cause the upregulation of a cytosolic machinery "inflammosome" to produce the pro-inflammatory cytokine IL-1β [6, 75 - 78].

Toll-like receptors (TLRs) are sensors of microbial and endogenous danger signals that are expressed and activated in innate immune cells and liver parenchymal cells, and induce signaling pathways of pro-inflammatory cytokines and chemokines. TLR-s in NASH are the important mediators of progression. *Pathogen- or damage-associated molecular patterns* (PAMPs or DAMPs) are TLR ligands inducing the activation of downstream signals. There are 10 TLRs indentified in humans, out of which TLR2, TLR4 and TLR9 are involved in the pathogenesis of NASH [4, 5]. *Kupffer cells* express TLR 2, 3, 4 and 9, which are responsive to lipopolysaccharide (LPS), and stimulation with LSP the cells produce ROS, inflammatory cytokines (TNFα, IL-1β, IL-6, IL-10, IL-12, IL-18 and cytokines stimulating fibrogenesis (TGFβ, MMPs PDGF). Kupffer cells sensing DAMPs are responsible for neutrophil granulocyte recruitment in the immune response. TLR-s are also expressed on hepatocytes, HSC-s, sinusoidal and biliary epithelial cells and hepatic dendritic cells as well [76, 77].

TLR2 is a receptor for glycolipids or lipoproteins in bacteria adhering to cell surface of monocytes, myeloid dendritic cells or mast cells [4].

TLR4 is located on the surfaces of Kupffer cells, monocytes, dendritic cells as well as B cells or mast cells. Pathogens from gut microbiota are important ligands for TLR4. Free cholesterol in hepatic stellate cells (HSCs) can result in increased TLR4 protein level similarly; cholesterol phagocytized by Kupffer cells induces their activation and TLR4 upregulation. This increased expression suppresses the endosomal-lysosomal degradation pathway of TLR4 and sensitizes cells to TGF-β- induced activation [4]. Thus, TLR4 is essential to NASH pathogenesis being a potent activator of innate immunity when it is stimulated by bacterial LSP. Disrupted intestinal epithelial function in chronic liver disease results in endotoxin (LPS) translocation from the gut and contributes to the progression of NASII. TLR4 (and TLR9) on recognizing LSP and FFA-s, induces inflammasome activation and production of IL-1β in Kupffer cells. Saturated fatty acids (SFAs) induce hepatocyte apoptosis and DAMPs from dying hepatocytes, thereby results in inflammation [6].

TLR9 is located on ER or endosomes of plasmacytoid dendritic cells or B cells and a receptor for unmethylated CpG DNA particles released from bacteria. **DNA** can act as DAMPs *via* their activation of TLR9. Mitochondria are rich of DAMPs and their signaling molecule, such as **ATP** can induce inflammosome activation. **HMGB**1 also is a nuclear protein that has been recognized as DAMP secreted by injured parenchymal cells [79, 80]. Endothelial cells have TLR9 receptors for DAMPs. Fibrogenesis in NASH may also be linked to TLRs. TLR signaling activates NF-κB, which upregulates the profibrogenic TGFβ [81].

Th17 Response

Th17 cells as a subset of effector Th cells secrete **IL-17,** function as both Th1 and Th2 cells, and represent a link between the innate and adaptive immune response. They are potent inducers of inflammation mostly mediated by neutrophils which are the cellular target of IL-17 [82, 83]. The combination of TGFβ and IL-6 promotes the induction of Th17 cells from naïve T cells and synergistically inhibits the generation of regulatory T cells, which suppress the inflammatory response [84]. Th17 cells secrete IL-17A, IL-17F, IL-21, IL-22 and TFNα, activate and mobilize neutrophils, act on hepatocytes to increase expression of inflammation associated genes, chemokines and CRP [85, 86]. The role of Th17 cells in the pathogenesis of NAFLD may be hypothesized by the increased plasma levels of IL-17 and liver infiltration with IL-17 positive cells that correlate with fibrosis severity [87]. IL-17 exacerbated FFA-induced steatosis in mice on high fat diet [84]. The presence of periportal and perivenular neutrophil infiltrate and increased levels of IL-6 in NASH also suggest a functional role for the Th17 response in the progression of NAFLD [88]. Similarly, the presence of IL-17 positive cells in portal inflammation was associated with ductular reaction (DR), suggesting that the Th17 response is implicated in fibrogenesis [72].

FIBROSIS, HEPATOCYTE BALLOONING, HEDGEHOG PATHWAY AND VITAMIN E IN NASH

Fibrosis in NASH is associated with ballooning of hepatocytes and reactivation of a developmental morphogenic signaling pathway, the hedgehog (Hh) [89 - 94].

Hepatocyte Ballooning

Lipotoxic liver cell injury is the key alteration in NASH. The main manifestation of lipotoxicity is *hepatocyte ballooning*, which is associated with accumulation of fat droplets, dilatation of cytoskeleton, abnormal protein production, and rendering hepatocytes vulnerable to apoptosis. Ballooned hepatocytes as injury-related cellular enlargement of hepatocytes represent a specific form of "cell degeneration". They contain dilated endoplasmic reticulum (ER) and ubiquitin aggregates, being keratin 8/18-negative ubiquitin-positive cells and located within fibrotic areas [90]. Ballooned hepatocytes exhibit signs of ER stress as key driver of NASH progression. When *toxic lipids* lead to c-Jun N terminal kinase (JNK) activation, an autocrine production and release of pro-fibrogenic soluble factors by ballooned hepatocytes occurs, that results in fibroblast differentiation into extracellular matrix component (EMC)-producing myofibroblasts. The numbers of ballooned hepatocytes correlate with the severity of fibrosis in NASH. Ballooned hepatocytes mean an increased risk for the development of fibrosis, and provide prognostic information regarding disease progression in NASH [91].

Lipotoxicity in ballooned hepatocytes is associated with JNK activation that induces expression of pleiotropic morphogens in the absence of cell death. Ballooned hepatocytes are not epiphenomena, but play a central role in the pathogenesis of NASH induced fibrosis, where they release the pro-fibrogenic factors, named as *hedgehog ligands* [92, 93].

Hedgehog Pathway

Hedgehog (Hh) is a developmental morphogenic signaling pathway. Hh ligands derived from primarily ballooned hepatocytes, activated ductular cells (DCs) and hepatic stellate cells (HSCs) mediate mesenchymal-epithelial interactions that regulate the development of many organs. Hh ligands are evolutionarily-conserved DAMP molecules that orchestrate regenerative responses in damaged tissues, stimulate stromal cells, such as myofibroblasts perpetuating fibrogenic repair [94].

Hh pathway becomes reactivated in many adults' organs during injury, to aid wound healing responses. Hh ligands promote remodeling in various tissues, thus lipotoxicity- associated liver injury also reactivates Hh signaling [95]. In hepatocytes, ER stress induces production of these ligands that provide paracrine profibrogenic signals to their microenvironment, neighboring Hh-responsive cells such as myofibroblasts. ER initially results in compensatory overexpression of viability factors but ultimately results in the production of microfolded proteins.

One member of Hh family is *Sonic Hedgehog* (SHh). Its target is a transmembrane-spanning cell surface receptor, *Patched* (Ptc). The interaction of ligands with Ptc inhibits basal Ptc-mediated suppression of **Smoothened** (Smo), the signaling component of Hh co-receptor. This initiates a signal activity leading to a cascade, that ultimately results in nuclear accumulation of glioblastoma family transcription factors (Gli1, 2,3), regulating the expression of Hh target genes encoding anti-apoptotic factors, viability, proliferation, migration and differentiation of Hh-responsive cells [95, 96].

Using stress-injured *Drosophila melanogaster* "undead cells", it was shown that ballooned cells produce SHh ligands [93, 94]. *Kakisaka et al.* [97] when modeled the "undead cell" concept, treated hepatocytes deficient in caspase 9 with toxic fatty acids. The lipotoxicity was associated with JNK activation and SHh expression in the absence of cell death. Ballooned hepatocytes in specimens from NASH patients also exhibited reduced expression of caspase 9, which may be analogous to the "undead cells" in *Drosophila melanogaster* model [98, 99] (Fig. **2**).

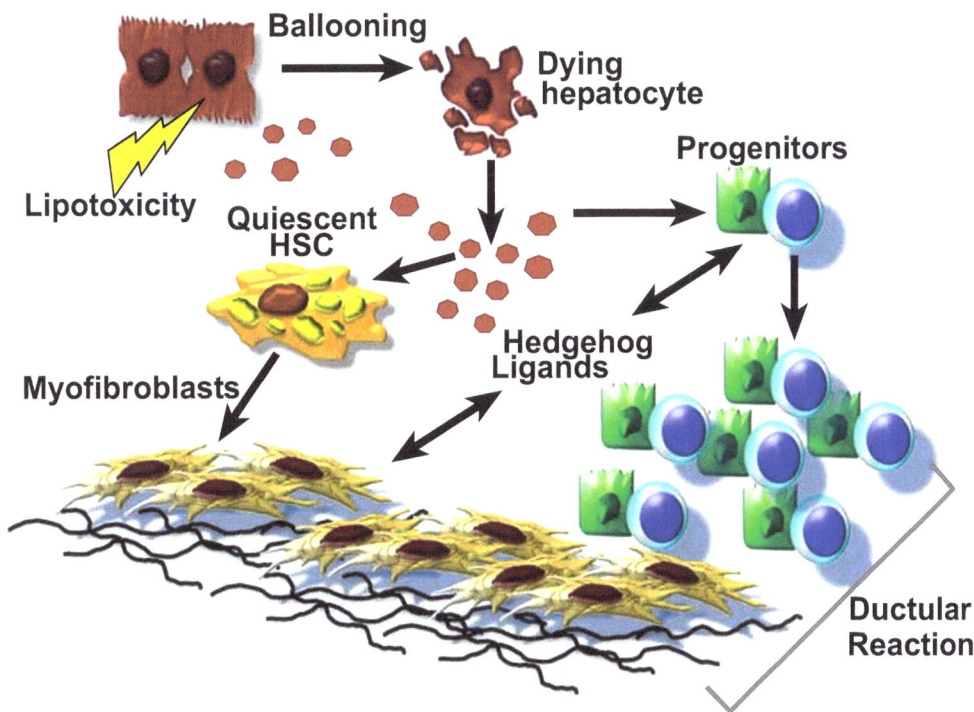

Fig. (2). Model of Hedgehod-mediated, deregulated fibrogenic repair in NASH after Guy *et al.* [99].

Ballooned hepatocytes are Gli2 negative, that is not Hh-responsive, but release Hh ligands, enriching the microenvironment with these factors, that stimulate the overgrowth of Hh responsive stromal cells. SHh functions as autocrine viability factor for cultured myofibroblasts. Expansion of fibrosis stage correlates with the extent of apoptosis and ballooning. Hh signal modulates growth factor actions (and *vice versa*) in Hh-responsive cells. The injury-related induction of Hh ligands can be regarded as a general regenerative mechanism. In normal liver, quiescent HSC-s (Q-HSC) silence Hh signals *via* Hh interactive protein (Hip). In liver injury, Hip production falls and Hh ligands become abundant, resulting in the formation of myofibroblasts from Q-HSC-s. The ligand-receptor interaction results in the nuclear accumulation of glioblastoma family transcription factors (gli1, gli2, gli3), which regulate the expression of Hh target genes, that control viability, proliferation, migration and differentiation of Hh-responsive cells [93, 99]. The level of Hh pathway activity parallels the severity of ballooning, inflammation and fibrosis in NASH patients [98]. Myofibroblastic cells and hepatic progenitor cells (HPCs) express receptors for Hh ligands, so that they are Hh responsive. Thus, HPCs, ballooned hepatocytes, myofibroblasts and reactive ductular cells along hedgehog pathway do play pivotal roles in hepatic regeneration and in the pathogenesis of fibrosis and ultimately cirrhosis in NASH [93, 99].

Vitamin E

Sanyal *et al.* in a clinical trial with pioglitazone and vitamin E (PIVENS) demonstrated that, compared to placebo, vitamin E therapy improved steatosis, lobular inflammation and hepatocyte ballooning in patients with NASH [100]. Recently, Guy *et al.* evaluated samples from vitamin E and placebo treatment groups from this trial, and showed that a greater decrease in SHh positive cells was found in responder as compared to nonresponders. Vitamin E therapy decreased the number of SHh positive hepatocytes in both responders and nonresponders, but a greater improvement in liver enzymes and lower number of SHh positive cells was seen in responders. Improvement in NASH was associated with decreased Hh pathway activity as assessed by number of SHh positive hepatocytes [99]. Thus, vitamin E can prevent oxidative stress associated with JNK activation, resulting in inhibition of SHh autocrine surviving signaling with deletion of ballooned hepatocytes. As a matter of fact vitamin E also reduced SHh-positive cells in nonresponders, suggesting that other unrelated mechanism may also contribute to tissue injury in NASH (Fig. **3** and **4**) [95].

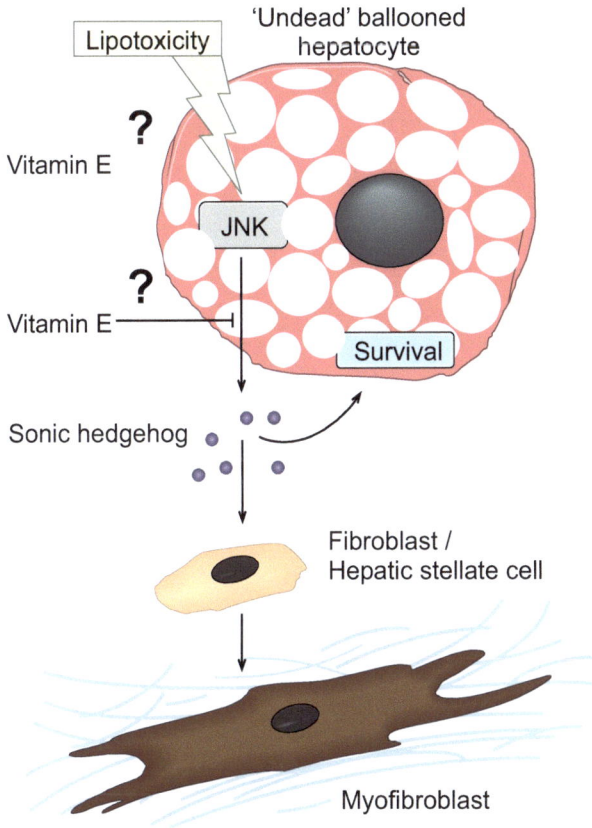

Fig. (3). Hedgehod pathway activation and vitamin E in NASH after Hirsova and Gores [95].

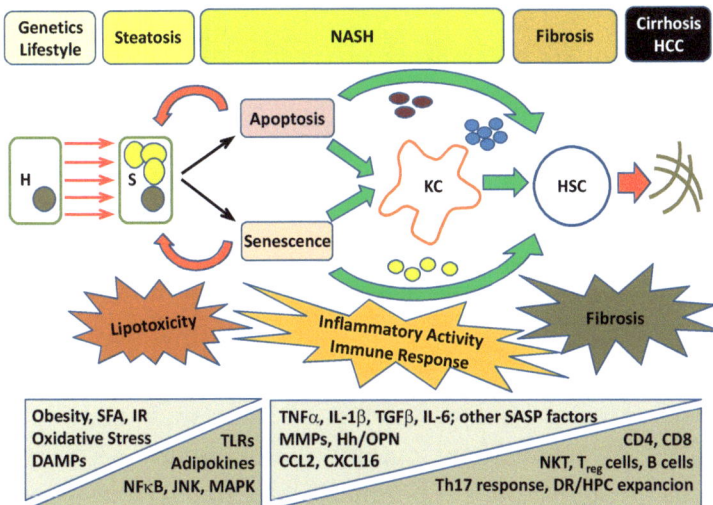

Fig. (4). The conception of NASH development according to Peverill *et al.* [5].

JNK activation by toxic lipids leads Sonic Hedgehog (SHh) production in ballooned hepatocytes. Released SHh acts through the autocrine pathway as a survival factor for "undead" ballooned hepatocytes and, through the paracrine mechanisms, induces fibroblast differentiation into extracellular matrix-producing myofibroblasts. Vitamin E decreases the amount of SHh in NASH by an unknown mechanism.

Multiple parallel metabolic hits lead to cellular damage, through a process called "lipotoxicity", oxidative stress driven by the metabolites of saturated fatty acids (SFA) (5). Injured hepatocytes release damage associated molecular patterns (DAMPs) that initiate an inflammatory response, *via* toll-like receptors (TLRs), and activate pro-inflammatory signaling pathways, increased adipokine levels. Hepatocytes undergo necrosis, apoptosis and senescence. Innate immune response develops with the activation of the inflammasome and the release of pro-inflammatory and pro-fibrogenic cytokines and ligands for *e.g.* Hedgehog (Hh), and osteopontin (OPN). Hepatic stellate cells (HSCs) produce extracellular matrix components leading to fibrosis, cirrhosis and HCC. Engulfment of apoptotic bodies and factors produced by senescent cells (adopting a "senescence-associated secretory phenotype" (SASP) also influences HSC activity. The activated Kupffer cells (KCs) and the pro-inflammatory microenvironment, initiate an adaptive immune response, representing a Th17 response. The chronic portal inflammatory infiltrate is accompanied by ductular reaction (DR) and hepatic progenitor cell (HPC) expansion.

SUMMARY

Hepatocytes are affected by lifestyle factors (diet and obesity) and genetic predispositions resulting in insulin resistance and steatosis. These multiple parallel metabolic hits lead to cellular damage, through a process called "lipotoxicity", an oxidative stress driven by the metabolites of saturated fatty acids. Injured hepatocytes release damage associated molecular patterns (DAMPs) that initiate an inflammatory response, *via* toll-like receptors and activated pro-inflammatory signaling pathways, and increased adipokine levels. Hepatocytes undergo necrosis, apoptosis and senescence, which are important to disease progression. Recruitment of Kupffer cells and other components of the innate immune response occur with activation of the inflammasome and the release of pro-inflammatory and pro-fibrogenic cytokines and ligand (*e.g.* Hedgehog). Hepatic stellate cells are activated and produce extracellular matrix components, leading to fibrosis, cirrhosis and its complications for *e.g.* HCC. Engulfment of apoptotic bodies and factors produced by senescent cells (adopting a "senescence-associated secretory phenotype") also influences HSC activity. The activity of Kupffer cells promotes a pro-inflammatory microenvironment that initiates an adaptive immune response, representing a Th17 response. The chronic portal inflammatory infiltrate is accompanied by ductular reaction and hepatic progenitor cell expansion. Ballooning of hepatocytes and reactivation of a developmental morphogenic signaling pathway, the hedgehog, are also associated with fibrosis that represents an imbalance of tissue damage and repair in NASH.

CONFLICT OF INTEREST

The author confirms that author has no conflict of interest to declare for this publication.

ACKNOWLEDGEMENTS

Declared none.

REFERENCES

[1]   Day CP, James OF. Steatohepatitis: a tale of two hits? Gastroenterology 1998; 114(4): 842-5.
        [http://dx.doi.org/10.1016/S0016-5085(98)70599-2] [PMID: 9547102]

[2]   Tilg H, Moschen AR. Evolution of inflammation in nonalcoholic fatty liver disease: the multiple parallel hits hypothesis. Hepatology 2010; 52(5): 1836-46.
        [http://dx.doi.org/10.1002/hep.24001] [PMID: 21038418]

[3]   Tiniakos DG, Vos MB, Brunt EM. Nonalcoholic fatty liver disease: pathology and pathogenesis. Annu Rev Pathol 2010; 5: 145-71.
        [http://dx.doi.org/10.1146/annurev-pathol-121808-102132] [PMID: 20078219]

[4]   Takaki A, Kawai D, Yamamoto K. Multiple hits, including oxidative stress, as pathogenesis and treatment target in non-alcoholic steatohepatitis (NASH). Int J Mol Sci 2013; 14(10): 20704-28.
        [http://dx.doi.org/10.3390/ijms141020704] [PMID: 24132155]

[5]   Peverill W, Powell LW, Skoien R. Evolving concepts in the pathogenesis of NASH: beyond steatosis and inflammation. Int J Mol Sci 2014; 15(5): 8591-638.
        [http://dx.doi.org/10.3390/ijms15058591] [PMID: 24830559]

[6]   Csak T, Ganz M, Pespisa J, Kodys K, Doldaniuc A, Szabo G. Fatty acids and endotoxin activate inflammasome in hepatocytes which release danger signals to activate immune cells in steatohepatitis. Hepatology 2011; 54: 133-44.
        [http://dx.doi.org/10.1002/hep.24341] [PMID: 21488066]

[7]   Pessayre D. Role of mitochondria in non-alcoholic fatty liver disease. J Gastroenterol Hepatol 2007; 22 (Suppl. 1): S20-7.
        [http://dx.doi.org/10.1111/j.1440-1746.2006.04640.x] [PMID: 17567459]

[8]   Novo E, Busletta C, Bonzo LV, *et al.* Intracellular reactive oxygen species are required for directional migration of resident and bone marrow-derived hepatic pro-fibrogenic cells. J Hepatol 2011; 54(5): 964-74.
        [http://dx.doi.org/10.1016/j.jhep.2010.09.022] [PMID: 21145826]

[9]   Byrne CD, Olufadi R, Bruce KD, Cagampang FR, Ahmed MH. Metabolic disturbances in non-alcoholic fatty liver disease. Clin Sci 2009; 116(7): 539-64.
[http://dx.doi.org/10.1042/CS20080253] [PMID: 19243311]

[10]   Lewis GF, Carpentier A, Adeli K, Giacca A. Disordered fat storage and mobilization in the pathogenesis of insulin resistance and type 2 diabetes. Endocr Rev 2002; 23(2): 201-29.
[http://dx.doi.org/10.1210/edrv.23.2.0461] [PMID: 11943743]

[11]   Zivkovic AM, German JB, Sanyal AJ. Comparative review of diets for the metabolic syndrome: implications for nonalcoholic fatty liver disease. Am J Clin Nutr 2007; 86(2): 285-300.
[PMID: 17684197]

[12]   Lo CJ, Chiu KC, Fu M, Lo R, Helton S. Fish oil decreases macrophage tumor necrosis factor gene transcription by altering the NF kappa B activity. J Surg Res 1999; 82(2): 216-21.
[http://dx.doi.org/10.1006/jsre.1998.5524] [PMID: 10090832]

[13]   Nishimaki-Mogami T, Yao Z, Fujimori K. Inhibition of phosphatidylcholine synthesis *via* the phosphatidylethanolamine methylation pathway impairs incorporation of bulk lipids into VLDL in cultured rat hepatocytes. J Lipid Res 2002; 43(7): 1035-45.
[http://dx.doi.org/10.1194/jlr.M100354-JLR200] [PMID: 12091487]

[14]   Abu-Elheiga L, Brinkley WR, Zhong L, Chirala SS, Woldegiorgis G, Wakil SJ. The subcellular localization of acetyl-CoA carboxylase 2. Proc Natl Acad Sci USA 2000; 97(4): 1444-9.
[http://dx.doi.org/10.1073/pnas.97.4.1444] [PMID: 10677481]

[15]   Chakravarthy MV, Pan Z, Zhu Y, *et al.* New hepatic fat activates PPARalpha to maintain glucose, lipid, and cholesterol homeostasis. Cell Metab 2005; 1(5): 309-22.
[http://dx.doi.org/10.1016/j.cmet.2005.04.002] [PMID: 16054078]

[16]   Yamaguchi K, Yang L, McCall S, *et al.* Diacylglycerol acyltranferase 1 anti-sense oligonucleotides reduce hepatic fibrosis in mice with nonalcoholic steatohepatitis. Hepatology 2008; 47(2): 625-35.
[http://dx.doi.org/10.1002/hep.21988] [PMID: 18000880]

[17]   Shimomura I, Shimano H, Korn BS, Bashmakov Y, Horton JD. Nuclear sterol regulatory element-binding proteins activate genes responsible for the entire program of unsaturated fatty acid biosynthesis in transgenic mouse liver. J Biol Chem 1998; 273(52): 35299-306.
[http://dx.doi.org/10.1074/jbc.273.52.35299] [PMID: 9857071]

[18]   Li J, Takaishi K, Cook W, McCorkle SK, Unger RH. Insig-1 brakes lipogenesis in adipocytes and inhibits differentiation of preadipocytes. Proc Natl Acad Sci USA 2003; 100(16): 9476-81.
[http://dx.doi.org/10.1073/pnas.1133426100] [PMID: 12869692]

[19]   Clement S, Krause U, Desmedt F, *et al.* The lipid phosphatase SHIP2 controls insulin sensitivity. Nature 2001; 409: 92-7.

[20]   Vinciguerra M, Foti M. PTEN and SHIP2 phosphoinositide phosphatases as negative regulators of insulin signalling. Arch Physiol Biochem 2006; 112(2): 89-104.
[http://dx.doi.org/10.1080/13813450600711359] [PMID: 16931451]

[21]   Tang X, Powelka AM, Soriano NA, Czech MP, Guilherme A. PTEN, but not SHIP2, suppresses insulin signaling through the phosphatidylinositol 3-kinase/Akt pathway in 3T3-L1 adipocytes. J Biol Chem 2005; 280(23): 22523-9.
[http://dx.doi.org/10.1074/jbc.M501949200] [PMID: 15824124]

[22]   Watanabe S, Horie Y, Kataoka E, *et al.* Non-alcoholic steatohepatitis and hepatocellular carcinoma: lessons from hepatocyte-specific phosphatase and tensin homolog (PTEN)-deficient mice. J Gastroenterol Hepatol 2007; 22 (Suppl. 1): S96-S100.
[http://dx.doi.org/10.1111/j.1440-1746.2006.04665.x] [PMID: 17567478]

[23]   Vinciguerra M, Veyrat-Durebex C, Moukil MA, Rubbia-Brandt L, Rohner-Jeanrenaud F, Foti M. PTEN down-regulation by unsaturated fatty acids triggers hepatic steatosis via an NF-kappaBp65/mTOR-dependent mechanism. Gastroenterology 2008; 134(1): 268-80.
[http://dx.doi.org/10.1053/j.gastro.2007.10.010] [PMID: 18166358]

[24]   Takano A, Usui I, Haruta T, *et al.* Mammalian target of rapamycin pathway regulates insulin signaling *via* subcellular redistribution of insulin receptor substrate 1 and integrates nutritional signals and metabolic signals of insulin. Mol Cell Biol 2001; 21(15): 5050-62.
[http://dx.doi.org/10.1128/MCB.21.15.5050-5062.2001] [PMID: 11438661]

[25]   Mordier S, Iynedjian PB. Activation of mammalian target of rapamycin complex 1 and insulin resistance induced by palmitate in hepatocytes. Biochem Biophys Res Commun 2007; 362(1): 206-11.
[http://dx.doi.org/10.1016/j.bbrc.2007.08.004] [PMID: 17698034]

[26]   Dentin R, Benhamed F, Pégorier JP, *et al.* Polyunsaturated fatty acids suppress glycolytic and lipogenic genes through the inhibition of ChREBP nuclear protein translocation. J Clin Invest 2005; 115(10): 2843-54.
[http://dx.doi.org/10.1172/JCI25256] [PMID: 16184193]

[27]   Chen G, Liang G, Ou J, Goldstein JL, Brown MS. Central role for liver X receptor in insulin-mediated activation of Srebp-1c transcription and stimulation of fatty acid synthesis in liver. Proc Natl Acad Sci USA 2004; 101(31): 11245-50.
[http://dx.doi.org/10.1073/pnas.0404297101] [PMID: 15266058]

[28]   Romeo S, Kozlitina J, Xing C, *et al.* Genetic variation in PNPLA3 confers susceptibility to nonalcoholic fatty liver disease. Nat Genet 2008; 40(12): 1461-5.
[http://dx.doi.org/10.1038/ng.257] [PMID: 18820647]

[29]   Kawaguchi T, Sumida Y, Umemura A, *et al.* Genetic polymorphisms of the human PNPLA3 gene are strongly associated with severity of non-alcoholic fatty liver disease in Japanese. PLoS One 2012; 7(6): e38322.
[http://dx.doi.org/10.1371/journal.pone.0038322] [PMID: 22719876]

[30]   Qiao A, Liang J, Ke Y, *et al.* Mouse patatin-like phospholipase domain-containing 3 influences systemic lipid and glucose homeostasis. Hepatology 2011; 54(2): 509-21.
[http://dx.doi.org/10.1002/hep.24402] [PMID: 21547936]

[31]   Burdge GC, Hanson MA, Slater-Jefferies JL, Lillycrop KA. Epigenetic regulation of transcription: a mechanism for inducing variations in phenotype (fetal programming) by differences in nutrition during early life? Br J Nutr 2007; 97(6): 1036-46.
[http://dx.doi.org/10.1017/S0007114507682920] [PMID: 17381976]

[32]   Burdge GC, Slater-Jefferies J, Torrens C, Phillips ES, Hanson MA, Lillycrop KA. Dietary protein restriction of pregnant rats in the F0 generation induces altered methylation of hepatic gene promoters in the adult male offspring in the F1 and F2 generations. Br J Nutr 2007; 97(3): 435-9.
[http://dx.doi.org/10.1017/S0007114507352392] [PMID: 17313703]

[33]   Bruce KD, Cagampang FR, Cagampang FR, Felino R. Epigenetic priming of the metabolic syndrome. Toxicol Mech Methods 2011; 21(4): 353-61.
[http://dx.doi.org/10.3109/15376516.2011.559370] [PMID: 21495873]

[34]   Yamauchi T, Kamon J, Minokoshi Y, *et al.* Adiponectin stimulates glucose utilization and fatty-acid oxidation by activating AMP-activated protein kinase. Nat Med 2002; 8(11): 1288-95.
[http://dx.doi.org/10.1038/nm788] [PMID: 12368907]

[35]   Hui JM, Hodge A, Farrell GC, Kench JG, Kriketos A, George J. Beyond insulin resistance in NASH: TNF-α or adiponectin? Hepatology 2004; 40(1): 46-54.
[http://dx.doi.org/10.1002/hep.20280] [PMID: 15239085]

[36] Polyzos SA, Toulis KA, Goulis DG, Zavos C, Kountouras J. Serum total adiponectin in nonalcoholic fatty liver disease: a systematic review and meta-analysis. Metabolism 2011; 60(3): 313-26.
[http://dx.doi.org/10.1016/j.metabol.2010.09.003] [PMID: 21040935]

[37] Carbone F, La Rocca C, Matarese G. Immunological functions of leptin and adiponectin. Biochimie 2012; 94(10): 2082-8.
[http://dx.doi.org/10.1016/j.biochi.2012.05.018] [PMID: 22750129]

[38] Lemoine M, Ratziu V, Kim M, *et al.* Serum adipokine levels predictive of liver injury in non-alcoholic fatty liver disease. Liver Int 2009; 29(9): 1431-8.
[http://dx.doi.org/10.1111/j.1478-3231.2009.02022.x] [PMID: 19422483]

[39] Han MS, Park SY, Shinzawa K, *et al.* Lysophosphatidylcholine as a death effector in the lipoapoptosis of hepatocytes. J Lipid Res 2008; 49(1): 84-97.
[http://dx.doi.org/10.1194/jlr.M700184-JLR200] [PMID: 17951222]

[40] OBrien J, Powell LW. Non-alcoholic fatty liver disease: is iron relevant? Hepatol Int 2012; 6(1): 332-41.
[http://dx.doi.org/10.1007/s12072-011-9304-9] [PMID: 22020821]

[41] George DK, Goldwurm S, MacDonald GA, *et al.* Increased hepatic iron concentration in nonalcoholic steatohepatitis is associated with increased fibrosis. Gastroenterology 1998; 114(2): 311-8.
[http://dx.doi.org/10.1016/S0016-5085(98)70482-2] [PMID: 9453491]

[42] Bonkovsky HL, Jawaid Q, Tortorelli K, *et al.* Non-alcoholic steatohepatitis and iron: increased prevalence of mutations of the HFE gene in non-alcoholic steatohepatitis. J Hepatol 1999; 31(3): 421-9.
[http://dx.doi.org/10.1016/S0168-8278(99)80032-4] [PMID: 10488699]

[43] Hernaez R, Yeung E, Clark JM, Kowdley KV, Brancati FL, Kao WH. Hemochromatosis gene and nonalcoholic fatty liver disease: a systematic review and meta-analysis. J Hepatol 2011; 55(5): 1079-85.
[http://dx.doi.org/10.1016/j.jhep.2011.02.013] [PMID: 21354231]

[44] Nelson JE, Wilson L, Brunt EM, *et al.* Relationship between the pattern of hepatic iron deposition and histological severity in nonalcoholic fatty liver disease. Hepatology 2011; 53(2): 448-57.
[http://dx.doi.org/10.1002/hep.24038] [PMID: 21274866]

[45] Yoneda M, Nozaki Y, Endo H, *et al.* Serum ferritin is a clinical biomarker in Japanese patients with nonalcoholic steatohepatitis (NASH) independent of HFE gene mutation. Dig Dis Sci 2010; 55(3): 808-14.
[http://dx.doi.org/10.1007/s10620-009-0771-y] [PMID: 19267193]

[46] van de Wier B, Balk JM, Haenen GR, *et al.* Elevated citrate levels in non-alcoholic fatty liver disease: the potential of citrate to promote radical production. FEBS Lett 2013; 587(15): 2461-6.
[http://dx.doi.org/10.1016/j.febslet.2013.06.019] [PMID: 23792160]

[47] Rolo AP, Teodoro JS, Palmeira CM. Role of oxidative stress in the pathogenesis of nonalcoholic steatohepatitis. Free Radic Biol Med 2012; 52(1): 59-69.
[http://dx.doi.org/10.1016/j.freeradbiomed.2011.10.003] [PMID: 22064361]

[48] Hernández-Gea V, Hilscher M, Rozenfeld R, *et al.* Endoplasmic reticulum stress induces fibrogenic activity in hepatic stellate cells through autophagy. J Hepatol 2013; 59(1): 98-104.
[http://dx.doi.org/10.1016/j.jhep.2013.02.016] [PMID: 23485523]

[49] Hernández-Gea V, Ghiassi-Nejad Z, Rozenfeld R, *et al.* Autophagy releases lipid that promotes fibrogenesis by activated hepatic stellate cells in mice and in human tissues. Gastroenterology 2012; 142(4): 938-46.
[http://dx.doi.org/10.1053/j.gastro.2011.12.044] [PMID: 22240484]

[50]   Gregor MG, Hotamisligil GS. Adipocyte stress: The endoplasmic reticulum and metabolic disease. J Lipid Res 2007; 48(9): 1905-14.

[51]   Targher G, Bertolini L, Rodella S, *et al.* Associations between plasma adiponectin concentrations and liver histology in patients with nonalcoholic fatty liver disease. Clin Endocrinol (Oxf) 2006; 64(6): 679-83.
[http://dx.doi.org/10.1111/j.1365-2265.2006.02527.x] [PMID: 16712671]

[52]   Tilg H, Moschen AR. Inflammatory mechanisms in the regulation of insulin resistance. Mol Med 2008; 14(3-4): 222-31.
[http://dx.doi.org/10.2119/2007-00119.Tilg] [PMID: 18235842]

[53]   Ron D. Translational control in the endoplasmic reticulum stress response. J Clin Invest 2002; 110(10): 1383-8.
[http://dx.doi.org/10.1172/JCI0216784] [PMID: 12438433]

[54]   Tilg H. Adipocytokines in nonalcoholic fatty liver disease: key players regulating steatosis, inflammation and fibrosis. Curr Pharm Des 2010; 16(17): 1893-5.
[http://dx.doi.org/10.2174/138161210791208929] [PMID: 20370678]

[55]   Feldstein AE, Canbay A, Angulo P, *et al.* Hepatocyte apoptosis and fas expression are prominent features of human nonalcoholic steatohepatitis. Gastroenterology 2003; 125(2): 437-43.
[http://dx.doi.org/10.1016/S0016-5085(03)00907-7] [PMID: 12891546]

[56]   Jaeschke H, Gujral JS, Bajt ML. Apoptosis and necrosis in liver disease. Liver Int 2004; 24(2): 85-9.
[http://dx.doi.org/10.1111/j.1478-3231.2004.0906.x] [PMID: 15078470]

[57]   Malhi H, Gores GJ, Lemasters JJ. Apoptosis and necrosis in the liver: a tale of two deaths? Hepatology 2006; 43(2) (Suppl. 1): S31-44.
[http://dx.doi.org/10.1002/hep.21062] [PMID: 16447272]

[58]   Malhi H, Barreyro FJ, Isomoto H, Bronk SF, Gores GJ. Free fatty acids sensitise hepatocytes to TRAIL mediated cytotoxicity. Gut 2007; 56(8): 1124-31.
[http://dx.doi.org/10.1136/gut.2006.118059] [PMID: 17470478]

[59]   Machado MV, Cortez-Pinto H. Cell death and nonalcoholic steatohepatitis: where is ballooning relevant? Expert Rev Gastroenterol Hepatol 2011; 5(2): 213-22.
[http://dx.doi.org/10.1586/egh.11.16] [PMID: 21476916]

[60]   Li Z, Berk M, McIntyre TM, Gores GJ, Feldstein AE. The lysosomal-mitochondrial axis in free fatty acid-induced hepatic lipotoxicity. Hepatology 2008; 47(5): 1495-503.
[http://dx.doi.org/10.1002/hep.22183] [PMID: 18220271]

[61]   Cazanave SC, Gores GJ. Mechanisms and clinical implications of hepatocyte lipoapoptosis. Clin Lipidol 2010; 5(1): 71-85.
[http://dx.doi.org/10.2217/clp.09.85] [PMID: 20368747]

[62]   Canbay A, Taimr P, Torok N, Higuchi H, Friedman S, Gores GJ. Apoptotic body engulfment by a human stellate cell line is profibrogenic. Lab Invest 2003; 83(5): 655-63.
[http://dx.doi.org/10.1097/01.LAB.0000069036.63405.5C] [PMID: 12746475]

[63]   Campisi J, dAdda di Fagagna F. Cellular senescence: when bad things happen to good cells. Nat Rev Mol Cell Biol 2007; 8(9): 729-40.
[http://dx.doi.org/10.1038/nrm2233] [PMID: 17667954]

[64]   Aravinthan A, Scarpini C, Tachtatzis P, *et al.* Hepatocyte senescence predicts progression in non-alcohol-related fatty liver disease. J Hepatol 2013; 58(3): 549-56.
[http://dx.doi.org/10.1016/j.jhep.2012.10.031] [PMID: 23142622]

[65]   Coppé JP, Desprez PY, Krtolica A, Campisi J. The senescence-associated secretory phenotype: the dark side of tumor suppression. Annu Rev Pathol 2010; 5: 99-118.
[http://dx.doi.org/10.1146/annurev-pathol-121808-102144] [PMID: 20078217]

[66]   Aravinthan A, Pietrosi G, Hoare M, *et al.* Hepatocyte expression of the senescence marker p21 is linked to fibrosis and an adverse liver-related outcome in alcohol-related liver disease. PLoS One 2013; 8(9): e72904.
[http://dx.doi.org/10.1371/journal.pone.0072904] [PMID: 24086266]

[67]   Krizhanovsky V, Yon M, Dickins RA, *et al.* Senescence of activated stellate cells limits liver fibrosis. Cell 2008; 134(4): 657-67.
[http://dx.doi.org/10.1016/j.cell.2008.06.049] [PMID: 18724938]

[68]   Richardson MM, Jonsson JR, Powell EE, *et al.* Progressive fibrosis in nonalcoholic steatohepatitis: association with altered regeneration and a ductular reaction. Gastroenterology 2007; 133(1): 80-90.
[http://dx.doi.org/10.1053/j.gastro.2007.05.012] [PMID: 17631134]

[69]   Zhan YT, An W. Roles of liver innate immune cells in nonalcoholic fatty liver disease. World J Gastroenterol 2010; 16(37): 4652-60.
[http://dx.doi.org/10.3748/wjg.v16.i37.4652] [PMID: 20872965]

[70]   Chen CJ, Kono H, Golenbock D, Reed G, Akira S, Rock KL. Identification of a key pathway required for the sterile inflammatory response triggered by dying cells. Nat Med 2007; 13(7): 851-6.
[http://dx.doi.org/10.1038/nm1603] [PMID: 17572686]

[71]   Bendelac A, Savage PB, Teyton L. The biology of NKT cells. Annu Rev Immunol 2007; 25: 297-336.
[http://dx.doi.org/10.1146/annurev.immunol.25.022106.141711] [PMID: 17150027]

[72]   Muhanna N, Horani A, Doron S, Safadi R. Lymphocyte-hepatic stellate cell proximity suggests a direct interaction. Clin Exp Immunol 2007; 148(2): 338-47.
[http://dx.doi.org/10.1111/j.1365-2249.2007.03353.x] [PMID: 17437422]

[73]   Gadd VL, Skoien R, Powell EE, *et al.* The portal inflammatory infiltrate and ductular reaction in human nonalcoholic fatty liver disease. Hepatology 2014; 59(4): 1393-405.
[http://dx.doi.org/10.1002/hep.26937] [PMID: 24254368]

[74]   Gao B, Seki E, Brenner DA, *et al.* Innate immunity in alcoholic liver disease. Am J Physiol Gastrointest Liver Physiol 2011; 300(4): G516-25.
[http://dx.doi.org/10.1152/ajpgi.00537.2010] [PMID: 21252049]

[75]   Davis BK, Wen H, Ting JP. The inflammasome NLRs in immunity, inflammation, and associated diseases. Annu Rev Immunol 2011; 29: 707-35.
[http://dx.doi.org/10.1146/annurev-immunol-031210-101405] [PMID: 21219188]

[76]   Silva MT. Secondary necrosis: the natural outcome of the complete apoptotic program. FEBS Lett 2010; 584(22): 4491-9.
[http://dx.doi.org/10.1016/j.febslet.2010.10.046] [PMID: 20974143]

[77]   Brenner DA, Seki E, Taura K, *et al.* Non-alcoholic steatohepatitis-induced fibrosis: Toll-like receptors, reactive oxygen species and Jun N-terminal kinase. Hepatol Res 2011; 41(7): 683-6.
[http://dx.doi.org/10.1111/j.1872-034X.2011.00814.x] [PMID: 21711427]

[78]   Rivera CA, Adegboyega P, van Rooijen N, Tagalicud A, Allman M, Wallace M. Toll-like receptor-4 signaling and Kupffer cells play pivotal roles in the pathogenesis of non-alcoholic steatohepatitis. J Hepatol 2007; 47(4): 571-9.
[http://dx.doi.org/10.1016/j.jhep.2007.04.019] [PMID: 17644211]

[79]   Tsung A, Klune JR, Zhang X, *et al.* HMGB1 release induced by liver ischemia involves Toll-like receptor 4 dependent reactive oxygen species production and calcium-mediated signaling. J Exp Med 2007; 204(12): 2913-23.
       [http://dx.doi.org/10.1084/jem.20070247] [PMID: 17984303]

[80]   Stros M. HMGB proteins: Interactions with DNA and chromatin. Biochim Biophys Acta 2010; 1799: 101-13.

[81]   Seki E, De Minicis S, Osterreicher CH, *et al.* TLR4 enhances TGF-beta signaling and hepatic fibrosis. Nat Med 2007; 13(11): 1324-32.
       [http://dx.doi.org/10.1038/nm1663] [PMID: 17952090]

[82]   Bettelli E, Carrier Y, Gao W, *et al.* Reciprocal developmental pathways for the generation of pathogenic effector TH17 and regulatory T cells. Nature 2006; 441(7090): 235-8.
       [http://dx.doi.org/10.1038/nature04753] [PMID: 16648838]

[83]   Miossec P, Korn T, Kuchroo VK. Interleukin-17 and type 17 helper T cells. N Engl J Med 2009; 361(9): 888-98.
       [http://dx.doi.org/10.1056/NEJMra0707449] [PMID: 19710487]

[84]   Tang Y, Bian Z, Zhao L, *et al.* Interleukin-17 exacerbates hepatic steatosis and inflammation in non-alcoholic fatty liver disease. Clin Exp Immunol 2011; 166(2): 281-90.
       [http://dx.doi.org/10.1111/j.1365-2249.2011.04471.x] [PMID: 21985374]

[85]   Jones CE, Chan K. Interleukin-17 stimulates the expression of interleukin-8, growth-related oncogene-alpha, and granulocyte-colony-stimulating factor by human airway epithelial cells. Am J Respir Cell Mol Biol 2002; 26(6): 748-53.
       [http://dx.doi.org/10.1165/ajrcmb.26.6.4757] [PMID: 12034575]

[86]   Sparna T, Rétey J, Schmich K, *et al.* Genome-wide comparison between IL-17 and combined TNF-alpha/IL-17 induced genes in primary murine hepatocytes. BMC Genomics 2010; 11: 226.
       [http://dx.doi.org/10.1186/1471-2164-11-226] [PMID: 20374638]

[87]   Lemmers A, Moreno C, Gustot T, *et al.* The interleukin-17 pathway is involved in human alcoholic liver disease. Hepatology 2009; 49(2): 646-57.
       [http://dx.doi.org/10.1002/hep.22680] [PMID: 19177575]

[88]   Hammerich L, Heymann F, Tacke F. Role of IL-17 and Th17 cells in liver diseases. Clin Dev Immunol 2011; 345803.

[89]   Gramlich T, Kleiner DE. McCullogh. Pathologic features with fibrosis in nonalcoholic fatty liver disease. Hum Pathol 2004; 35: 196-9.
       [http://dx.doi.org/10.1016/j.humpath.2003.09.018] [PMID: 14991537]

[90]   Caldwell S, Ikura Y, Dias D, *et al.* Hepatocellular ballooning in NASH. J Hepatol 2010; 53(4): 719-23.
       [http://dx.doi.org/10.1016/j.jhep.2010.04.031] [PMID: 20624660]

[91]   Jung Y, Diehl AM. Non-alcoholic steatohepatitis pathogenesis: role of repair in regulating the disease progression. Dig Dis 2010; 28(1): 225-8.
       [http://dx.doi.org/10.1159/000282092] [PMID: 20460916]

[92]   Bohinc BN, Diehl AM. Mechanisms of disease progression in NASH: new paradigms. Clin Liver Dis 2012; 16(3): 549-65.
       [http://dx.doi.org/10.1016/j.cld.2012.05.002] [PMID: 22824480]

[94]   Rangwala F, Guy CD, Lu J, *et al.* Increased production of sonic hedgehog by ballooned hepatocytes. J Pathol 2011; 224(3): 401-10.
       [http://dx.doi.org/10.1002/path.2888] [PMID: 21547909]

[95]   Hirsova P, Gores GJ. Ballooned hepatocytes, undead cells, sonic hedgehog, and vitamin E: therapeutic implications for nonalcoholic steatohepatitis. Hepatology 2015; 61(1): 15-7.
[http://dx.doi.org/10.1002/hep.27279] [PMID: 24975580]

[96]   Briscoe J, Thérond PP. The mechanisms of Hedgehog signalling and its roles in development and disease. Nat Rev Mol Cell Biol 2013; 14(7): 416-29.
[http://dx.doi.org/10.1038/nrm3598] [PMID: 23719536]

[97]   Kakisaka K, Cazanave SC, Werneburg NW, *et al.* A hedgehog survival pathway in undead lipotoxic hepatocytes. J Hepatol 2012; 57(4): 844-51.
[http://dx.doi.org/10.1016/j.jhep.2012.05.011] [PMID: 22641094]

[98]   Guy CD, Suzuki A, Zdanowicz M, *et al.* Hedgehog pathway activation parallels histologic severity of injury and fibrosis in human nonalcoholic fatty liver disease. Hepatology 2012; 55(6): 1711-21.
[http://dx.doi.org/10.1002/hep.25559] [PMID: 22213086]

[99]   Guy CD, Suzuki A, Abdelmalek MF, Burchette JL, Diehl AM. Treatment response in the PIVENS trial is associated with decreased Hedgehog pathway activity. Hepatology 2015; 61(1): 98-107.
[http://dx.doi.org/10.1002/hep.27235] [PMID: 24849310]

[100]   Sanyal AJ, Chalasani N, Kowdley KV, *et al.* Pioglitazone, vitamin E, or placebo for nonalcoholic steatohepatitis. N Engl J Med 2010; 362(18): 1675-85.
[http://dx.doi.org/10.1056/NEJMoa0907929] [PMID: 20427778]

CHAPTER 6

Metabolic Diseases and NAFLD

Tatjana Ábel[a,b,*]

[a] *Outpatient Department, Military Hospital, Budapest Hungary*

[b] *Faculty of Health Sciences, Semmelweis University, Budapest, Hungary*

Abstract: Non-alcoholic fatty liver disease (NAFLD) is one of the most common causes of elevated liver enzymes and chronic liver disease in the Western countries. NAFLD has been noted to be common in patients with obesity, hypertension, type 2 diabetes and atherogenic dyslipidemia. In the United States, it is estimated that NAFLD affects 20-30% of the general population. In patients with diabetes, the prevalence of NAFLD has been reported to be 70%. A high prevalence of NAFLD was found in patients with type 2 diabetes and obesity (90%). NAFLD is an independent predictor of future risk of cardiovascular diseases, and metabolic syndrome as well.

Keywords : Cardiovascular, Cholesterol, Diabetes, Dyslipidemia, HOMA-IR, Hypertension, Inflammation, Insulin resistance, Lipid disorder, Metabolic syndrome, Obesity, Triglyceride.

INTRODUCTION

NAFLD is one of the most prevalent hepatic diseases in the developed countries [1]. It affects approximately 20 to 30% of the population [2 - 4]. The prevalence of NAFLD, however, also depends on the ethnical group and on the presence of other diseases. It occurs in 5 to 40% of populations in Asian countries [5]. A study in the USA showed that NASH occurred at the highest rate among Hispanics (47%) and at the lowest rate in the black population (24%) [6].

The prevalence of NAFLD may even be 90% in obese people, and 70% in patients with diabetes [7, 8]. The results of two large European studies showed the prevalence of 42.6-69.5% for NAFLD in patients with type 2 diabetes mellitus [9, 10].

---

[*] **Corresponding author Tatjana Ábel:** Outpatient Department, Military Hospital, 1134 Budapest, Róbert Károly krt. 44., Hungary; E-mail: abelt@t-online.hu

Tatjana Ábel & Gabriella Lengyel (Eds.)
All rights reserved-© 2017 Bentham Science Publishers

Other metabolic diseases that constitute a part of the metabolic syndrome, such as hypertension or atherogenic dyslipidemia (hypercholesterolemia, hypertriglyceridemia, or a combination of these) can also be found more frequently, in 20 to 80% of patients with NAFLD [11].

In the developed countries cardiovascular (CV) diseases are the leading cause of mortality [12]. According to the report of the World Health Organization (WHO), 17.3 million people died as a consequence of CV diseases in 2008, which represented 30% of the total mortality in that year [13]. This number increased further to 2012, when 17.5 million people died due to CV diseases, representing already 31% of the total mortality [14].

Results published up to now showed that the presence of NAFLD increases the risk of both total mortality and mortality due to CV diseases [15 - 18].

On average, *NASH* occurs in approx. 2 to 3% of the population [19, 20]. A survey among patients with type 2 diabetes mellitus, however, showed a prevalence of 63-87% for NASH and 22-60% for moderate to severe fibrosis [21]. In the USA, NASH is currently the 3rd most common cause of liver transplantation after hepatitis C and alcoholic liver disease [22, 23]. It is estimated, however, that NASH may be the most frequent cause of liver transplantation between 2020 and 2025 [23].

OBESITY

Up to now, the results show a close correlation between obesity (mainly abdominal obesity due to increased visceral adipose tissue) and the elevated risk of developing and progressing NAFLD and NASH (Fig. **1**) [24 - 28]. Adipose tissue has been referred to for years as an endocrine organ that produces, among others, tissue-specific cytokines, so-called adipokines as well. These cytokines [*e.g.* adiponectin, leptin, tumor necrosis factor-alpha (TNF-α), interleukin-6 (IL-6), resistin] may influence the extent of insulin sensitivity, the decrease of which shows a close correlation with the increase in the risk of developing NAFLD [29]. In addition, the increased amount of free fatty acids (FFAs) released from the adipose tissue also has a decisive importance in the progression of hepatic lesion [30].

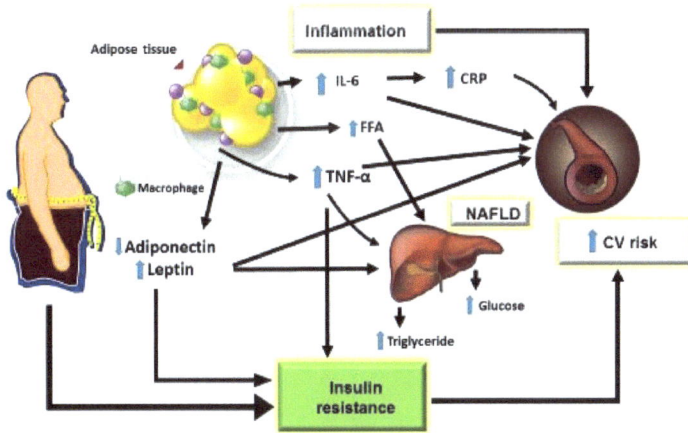

Fig. (1). Connection between abdominal obesity and NAFLD.

CRP = C-reactive protein; FFA = free fatty acids; IL = Interleukin; TNF-α = tumor necrosis factor alpha.

Several studies showed insulin resistance, *i.e.* an elevated value of homeostasis model assessment of insulin resistance (HOMA-IR) index exceeding 5.8 in non-diabetic overweight patients with NAFLD [31, 32].

In addition, results published up to now show a correlation between the diameter of adipocytes and the extent of hepatic lesion as well [33]. In the study of Wree *et al.* the data of 93 severely obese individuals (mean age 43 years; average BMI 52 kg/m^2) with NAFLD or NASH were compared before bariatric surgery and 6 weeks after the intervention. Also, a relationship has been demonstrated between increased adipocyte diameter and factors related to hepatic lesion such as lower adiponectin level, and higher levels of C-reactive protein (CRP), leptin, FFAs, transaminases and apolipoproteins [particularly apolipoprotein C-III (apo CIII)]. However, according to their results adipocyte cell diameter was found to be independent of BMI and gender as well, as demonstrated previously by O'Conell *et al.* [33, 34].

An approximately 5% reduction of body weight already mitigates the degree of steatosis and the concentrations of transaminases as well [35 - 37]. However, an approx. 10% reduction of body weight is often associated with a histological improvement and a moderated progression of hepatic impairment [35]. Nevertheless, a rapid reduction of body mass (24% in 8 weeks) may increase portal inflammation and the degree of fibrosis [38]. These results also demonstrate that the successful treatment of NAFLD relies on the gradual reduction of body weight.

TYPE 2 DIABETES

The number of diabetic patients was calculated to be 366 million worldwide in 2011, and according to the predictive estimations it will be 522 million until 2030 [39]. More than 90% of these patients have type 2 diabetes. Mortality due to CV diseases affects approximately two thirds of type 2 diabetic patients [40].

Similar risk factors and pathogenic mechanisms are shared by the development of NAFLD and type 2 diabetes [41]. The development of insulin resistance has a decisive role in the appearance of both of diseases [42].

Targher *et al.* found a higher prevalence of coronary, cerebrovascular and peripheral vascular disease in type 2 diabetic patients with NAFLD as compared to patients with no NAFLD [43]. NAFLD, however, showed a correlation not only with the macrovascular, but also with the microvascular complications of patients with type 2 diabetes [42, 44, 45]. For NAFLD a higher prevalence was also found in relation to microalbuminuria, chronic nephropathy and retinopathy in diabetic patients [42, 46, 47].

Not only the development of type 2 diabetes can be predicted by NAFLD, but type 2 diabetes may also increase the chance for developing NAFLD and even the degree of progression [42, 48 - 52]. The results of a study showed a considerably higher rate of developing NASH and severe hepatic fibrosis in patients with type 2 diabetes in comparison to non-diabetic patients [53].

As the results up to now have shown, the extent of steatosis and its progression can be reduced by changes in the lifestyle (diet, exercise, weight loss) as in the treatment of type 2 diabetes, and also through medication using insulin-sensitizing agents (metformin, pioglitazone) and newer agents, which cause no hypoglycemia (dipeptidyl-peptidase IV inhibitors, glucagon-like peptide-1 analogues) [54 - 62].

LIPID DISORDERS

Lipid disorders can be found in 70-80% of patients with NAFLD [63]. Due to developing NAFLD, there is an increased CV morbidity, which can be further increased by the appearance of hyperlipidemia.

In patients with NAFLD or NASH, triglyceride levels are often elevated, and HDL-cholesterol levels are decreased [64, 65]. The increase in triglycerides is secondary in the majority of cases, as VLDL concentration and size are increased during the development of NAFLD [66, 67]. The decrease of HDL-cholesterol occurs also secondarily, as the increased triglyceride concentration increases the cholesterol ester transfer protein (CETP)-mediated incorporation of triglycerides into the HDL-particle. These HDL particles, rich in triglyceride, are withdrawn from the circulation much more rapidly [68].

In the study of DeFilippis *et al.*, in addition to a rise in triglycerides and a decrease in HDL-C, an increased hepatic production of apoprotein B100 containing particles (large VLDL, VLDL, IDL) was observed [66]. Consequently, the production of cholesterol-rich LDL particles was also increased.

Statins used in hyperlipidemia have been shown in several studies to reduce the risk of CV diseases both in primary and in secondary prevention [69, 70]. In addition to their main effect, statins also possess a so-called pleiotropic activity such as endothelial dysfunction-reducing, anti-inflammatory, antioxidant, antiplatelet and anti-proliferative effects [71]. One of the potential side effects of statin therapy may be, however, an increase in hepatic transaminase enzymes. Nevertheless, in the majority of observations, the levels of transaminases showed a significant decrease due to statin therapy [72 - 75]. Introduction of statin therapy for patients with dyslipidemic NAFLD or NASH is recommended by the American Association for the Study of Liver Diseases, the American College of Gastroenterology and the American Gastroenterological Association [76].

In a prospective, non-randomized study of cholesterol-lowering ezetimibe therapy of a few patients (n=10), patients with NASH showed significant improvement in the levels of transaminases, GGT, LDL-cholesterol, HDL-cholesterol type IV collagen 7S and CRP [77]. Liver biopsies were performed before ezetimibe therapy and 6 months after it. An improved degree of fibrosis was detected in 6 of the 10 patients. In another study, also confirmed by liver biopsy, patients with NAFLD (n=45) received ezetimibe therapy (10 mg/day) for 24 months [78]. Ezetimibe therapy reduced the visceral adipose mass, the fasting insulin level, the HOMA index, the triglyceride, total cholesterol and LDL-cholesterol levels as well. In addition, the therapy significantly reduced serum ALT and CRP concentrations, too. Levels of type IV collagen 7S, adiponectin, leptin, and resistin also decreased upon ezetimibe therapy. Repeated liver biopsy showed also a significant decrease in the degree of steatosis (P= 0.0003) and the proportion of necro-inflammation (P=0.00456), while the degree of fibrosis showed no significant improvement (P=0.6547). In a retrospective study of our working group, combined ezetimibe/simvastatin therapy (n=19) or simvastatin monotherapy (n=26) for 6 months has significantly reduced, in addition to cholesterol levels, also ALT and AST values in patients with NAFLD, type 2 diabetes and hypercholesterolemia [79].

As for fibrate therapy, the results are controversial. Some observations found a reduced hepatic fat content upon fibrate therapy, others, however, showed no improvement during histological examination of the liver, although hepatic transaminase levels decreased [80 - 83].

HYPERTENSION

The relationship between NAFLD and hypertension has been studied, however, less than the correlation of NAFLD with diabetes, obesity or dyslipidemia. The prevalence of NAFLD in hypertensive patients was 49.5-57.5% [84, 85]. In the middle-aged and elderly, NAFLD has proven to be an independent risk factor in those with hypertension or high-normal systolic blood pressure values. In a population-based (n=3191), prospective, longitudinal study approximately three times higher chance was found for developing hypertension during the follow-up in those with fatty liver disease (FLD) as compared to patients with no FLD [86]. A relationship was also found between NAFLD and the development of left ventricle hypertrophy, ventricular dysfunction and cardiovascular dysautonomia as well [87 - 89].

In obese hypertensive patients NAFLD has proven to be a significant and independent CV risk factor [90 - 92]. In addition, studies were published where a relationship was found between hypertension and NAFLD also in lean individuals [93 - 95]. Study results of Aneni *et al.* showed at first a connection between prehypertension (PHT) and NAFLD, also in individuals with no other metabolic risk factors [95]. Based on this, it emerged that PHT may be considered as an early marker of NAFLD in individuals otherwise with a low risk of CV disease.

The exact mechanism of the relationship between NAFLD and hypertension is not known. It is supposed that the development of insulin resistance has a decisive importance in it [93, 96]. In the study of Fallo *et al.* patients with primary hypertension (n=80) were in part dippers (n=47), in part non-dippers (n=33) (Fallo 2008). The patients had neither diabetes nor hyperlipidemia, and they were not obese. NAFLD was found at a significantly higher rate in non-dipper patients as compared to dippers (81.8 *vs.* 40.4%, P<0.005). Insulin levels and HOMA index were significantly higher (P<0.001), while adiponectin concentrations were lower (P<0.001) in non-dippers as compared to dippers.

METABOLIC SYNDROME

Based on the results of the recent years, NAFLD is regarded as the hepatic manifestation of the metabolic syndrome [97, 98]. Metabolic syndrome entails a group of metabolic diseases/disorders which represent a CV risk. The newer definition of International Diabetes Federation (IDF) has modified the previous definition of metabolic syndrome (Tables **1** and **2**) [99]. In addition to the central obesity, two further abnormities are required for the presence of metabolic syndrome.

Table 1. Definition of the metabolic syndrome according to IDF [99].

Central obesity waist circumference - ethnicity specific (see Table **2**)
Plus any two:

Raised triglycerides
    > 150 mg/dL (1.7 mmol/L)
    Specific treatment for this lipid abnormality

Reduced HDL-cholesterol   < 40 mg/dL (1.03 mmol/L) in men   < 50 mg/dL (1.29 mmol/L) in women Specific treatment for this lipid abnormality

Raised blood pressure
    Systolic ≥ 130 mmHg
    Diastolic ≥ 85 mmHg
Treatment of previously diagnosed hypertension

Raised fasting plasma glucose
    Fasting plasma glucose ≥ 100 mg/dL (5.6 mmol/L)
    Previously diagnosed type 2 diabetes
    If above value is 5.6 mmol/L or 100 mg/dL, oral glucose tolerance test is strongly recommended, but the value does not signifies the presence of syndrome

Table 2. Ethnic-specific values for waist circumference [99].

Ethnic Group	**Waist Circumference** **(as Measure of Central Obesity)**
Europids* Men Women	≥ 94 cm (37 in) ≥ 80 cm (32 in)
South Asians Men Women	≥ 90 cm (35 in) ≥ 80 cm (32 in)
Chinese Men Women	≥ 90 cm (35 in) ≥ 80 cm (32 in)

(Table 2) contd.....

Ethnic Group	Waist Circumference (as Measure of Central Obesity)
Japanese Men Women	≥ 85 cm (34 in) ≥ 90 cm (35 in)
Ethnic South and Central Americans	Use South Asian recommendations until more specific data are available
Sub-Saharan Africans	Use European data until more specific data are available
Eastern Mediterranean and middle east (Arab) populations	Use European data until more specific data are available

*In USA, Adult Treatment Panel III values (102 cm male, 88 cm female) are likely to continue to be used for clinical purposes.

Metabolic abnormities found in metabolic syndrome showed a correlation with the development and progression of NAFLD, separately. NAFLD confirmed by liver biopsy occurred in 86% of patients with metabolic syndrome, while steatohepatitis and cirrhosis occurred in 24% and 2% of them respectively [100]. According to the recently published survey NAFLD can be considered as a predictor of developing metabolic syndrome [101].

CONCLUDING REMARKS

NAFLD is one of the most frequent hepatic diseases in the developed countries. It can be regarded as an independent risk factor of CV diseases. NAFLD is often associated with obesity, type 2 diabetes, atherogenic hyperlipidemia, and hypertension, *i.e.* with diseases belonging to the metabolic syndrome. Therefore, the spread of NAFLD and the diseases associated with it represents an ever increasing burden for health care and budget in these countries. The prevention and the treatment of NAFLD and its complications as early as possible have an outstanding importance.

CONFLICT OF INTEREST

The author confirms that author has no conflict of interest to declare for this publication.

ACKNOWLEDGEMENTS

Declared none.

REFERENCES

[1]   Kim NH, Park J, Kim SH, *et al.* Non-alcoholic fatty liver disease, metabolic syndrome and subclinical cardiovascular changes in the general population. Heart 2014; 100(12): 938-43.
       [http://dx.doi.org/10.1136/heartjnl-2013-305099] [PMID: 24721975]

[2]   Colicchio P, Tarantino G, del Genio F, *et al.* Non-alcoholic fatty liver disease in young adult severely obese non-diabetic patients in South Italy. Ann Nutr Metab 2005; 49(5): 289-95.
[http://dx.doi.org/10.1159/000087295] [PMID: 16088092]

[3]   Akbar DH, Kawther AH. Non-alcoholic fatty liver disease and metabolic syndrome: what we know and what we dont know. Med Sci Monit 2006; 12(1): RA23-6.
[PMID: 16369477]

[4]   Lazo M, Clark JM. The epidemiology of nonalcoholic fatty liver disease: a global perspective. Semin Liver Dis 2008; 28(4): 339-50.
[http://dx.doi.org/10.1055/s-0028-1091978] [PMID: 18956290]

[5]   Amarapurkar DN, Hashimoto E, Lesmana LA, Sollano JD, Chen PJ, Goh KL. How common is non-alcoholic fatty liver disease in the Asia-Pacific region and are there local differences? J Gastroenterol Hepatol 2007; 22(6): 788-93.
[http://dx.doi.org/10.1111/j.1440-1746.2007.05042.x] [PMID: 17565631]

[6]   Browning JD, Szczepaniak LS, Dobbins R, *et al.* Prevalence of hepatic steatosis in an urban population in the United States: impact of ethnicity. Hepatology 2004; 40(6): 1387-95.
[http://dx.doi.org/10.1002/hep.20466] [PMID: 15565570]

[7]   Gastaldelli A, Cusi K, Pettiti M, *et al.* Relationship between hepatic/visceral fat and hepatic insulin resistance in nondiabetic and type 2 diabetic subjects. Gastroenterology 2007; 133(2): 496-506.
[http://dx.doi.org/10.1053/j.gastro.2007.04.068] [PMID: 17681171]

[8]   Gaggini M, Morelli M, Buzzigoli E, DeFronzo RA, Bugianesi E, Gastaldelli A. Non-alcoholic fatty liver disease (NAFLD) and its connection with insulin resistance, dyslipidemia, atherosclerosis and coronary heart disease. Nutrients 2013; 5(5): 1544-60.
[http://dx.doi.org/10.3390/nu5051544] [PMID: 23666091]

[9]   Targher G, Bertolini L, Padovani R, *et al.* Prevalence of nonalcoholic fatty liver disease and its association with cardiovascular disease among type 2 diabetic patients. Diabetes Care 2007; 30(5): 1212-8.
[http://dx.doi.org/10.2337/dc06-2247] [PMID: 17277038]

[10]   Williamson RM, Price JF, Glancy S, *et al.* Prevalence of and risk factors for hepatic steatosis and nonalcoholic Fatty liver disease in people with type 2 diabetes: the Edinburgh Type 2 Diabetes Study. Diabetes Care 2011; 34(5): 1139-44.
[http://dx.doi.org/10.2337/dc10-2229] [PMID: 21478462]

[11]   Souza MR, Diniz MdeF, Medeiros-Filho JE, Araújo MS. Metabolic syndrome and risk factors for non-alcoholic fatty liver disease. Arq Gastroenterol 2012; 49(1): 89-96.
[http://dx.doi.org/10.1590/S0004-28032012000100015] [PMID: 22481692]

[12]   Ma X, Zhu S. Metabolic syndrome in the prevention of cardiovascular diseases and diabetes still a matter of debate? Eur J Clin Nutr 2013; 67(5): 518-21.
[http://dx.doi.org/10.1038/ejcn.2013.24] [PMID: 23403882]

[13]   Global atlas on cardiovascular disease prevention and control: policies, strategies and interventions 2011. http://www.who.int/cardiovascular_diseases/publications/atlas_cvd/

[14]   Cardiovascular diseases (CVDs). Key facts 2015. http://www.who.int/mediacentre/factsheets/fs317/en/

[15]   Blachier M, Leleu H, Peck-Radosavljevic M, Valla DC, Roudot-Thoraval F. The burden of liver disease in Europe: a review of available epidemiological data. J Hepatol 2013; 58(3): 593-608.
[http://dx.doi.org/10.1016/j.jhep.2012.12.005] [PMID: 23419824]

[16]   Oni ET, Agatston AS, Blaha MJ, *et al.* A systematic review: burden and severity of subclinical cardiovascular disease among those with nonalcoholic fatty liver; should we care? Atherosclerosis 2013; 230(2): 258-67.

[http://dx.doi.org/10.1016/j.atherosclerosis.2013.07.052] [PMID: 24075754]

[17]   Nestel PJ, Mensink RP. Perspective: nonalcoholic fatty liver disease and cardiovascular risk. Curr Opin Lipidol 2013; 24(1): 1-3.
       [http://dx.doi.org/10.1097/MOL.0b013e32835c0834] [PMID: 23298957]

[18]   Brea A, Puzo J. Non-alcoholic fatty liver disease and cardiovascular risk. Int J Cardiol 2013; 167(4): 1109-17.
       [http://dx.doi.org/10.1016/j.ijcard.2012.09.085] [PMID: 23141876]

[19]   Bellentani S, Scaglioni F, Marino M, Bedogni G. Epidemiology of non-alcoholic fatty liver disease. Dig Dis 2010; 28(1): 155-61.
       [http://dx.doi.org/10.1159/000282080] [PMID: 20460905]

[20]   Vernon G, Baranova A, Younossi ZM. Systematic review: the epidemiology and natural history of non-alcoholic fatty liver disease and non-alcoholic steatohepatitis in adults. Aliment Pharmacol Ther 2011; 34(3): 274-85.
       [http://dx.doi.org/10.1111/j.1365-2036.2011.04724.x] [PMID: 21623852]

[21]   Leite NC, Villela-Nogueira CA, Pannain VL, *et al.* Histopathological stages of nonalcoholic fatty liver disease in type 2 diabetes: prevalences and correlated factors. Liver Int 2011; 31(5): 700-6.
       [http://dx.doi.org/10.1111/j.1478-3231.2011.02482.x] [PMID: 21457442]

[22]   Charlton MR, Burns JM, Pedersen RA, Watt KD, Heimbach JK, Dierkhising RA. Frequency and outcomes of liver transplantation for nonalcoholic steatohepatitis in the United States. Gastroenterology 2011; 141(4): 1249-53.
       [http://dx.doi.org/10.1053/j.gastro.2011.06.061] [PMID: 21726509]

[23]   Rahimi RS, Landaverde C. Nonalcoholic fatty liver disease and the metabolic syndrome: clinical implications and treatment. Nutr Clin Pract 2013; 28(1): 40-51.
       [http://dx.doi.org/10.1177/0884533612470464] [PMID: 23286927]

[24]   Bettermann K, Hohensee T, Haybaeck J. Steatosis and steatohepatitis: complex disorders. Int J Mol Sci 2014; 15(6): 9924-44.
       [http://dx.doi.org/10.3390/ijms15069924] [PMID: 24897026]

[25]   van der Poorten D, Milner KL, Hui J, *et al.* Visceral fat: a key mediator of steatohepatitis in metabolic liver disease. Hepatology 2008; 48(2): 449-57.
       [http://dx.doi.org/10.1002/hep.22350] [PMID: 18627003]

[26]   Beasley LE, Koster A, Newman AB, *et al.* Inflammation and race and gender differences in computerized tomography-measured adipose depots. Obesity (Silver Spring) 2009; 17(5): 1062-9.
       [http://dx.doi.org/10.1038/oby.2008.627] [PMID: 19165157]

[27]   Gabriely I, Ma XH, Yang XM, *et al.* Removal of visceral fat prevents insulin resistance and glucose intolerance of aging: an adipokine-mediated process? Diabetes 2002; 51(10): 2951-8.
       [http://dx.doi.org/10.2337/diabetes.51.10.2951] [PMID: 12351432]

[28]   Dietrich P, Hellerbrand C. Non-alcoholic fatty liver disease, obesity and the metabolic syndrome. Best Pract Res Clin Gastroenterol 2014; 28(4): 637-53.
       [http://dx.doi.org/10.1016/j.bpg.2014.07.008] [PMID: 25194181]

[29]   Bugianesi E, McCullough AJ, Marchesini G. Insulin resistance: a metabolic pathway to chronic liver disease. Hepatology 2005; 42(5): 987-1000.
       [http://dx.doi.org/10.1002/hep.20920] [PMID: 16250043]

[30]   Neuschwander-Tetri BA. Hepatic lipotoxicity and the pathogenesis of nonalcoholic steatohepatitis: the central role of nontriglyceride fatty acid metabolites. Hepatology 2010; 52(2): 774-88.
       [http://dx.doi.org/10.1002/hep.23719] [PMID: 20683968]

[31]   Boza C, Riquelme A, Ibañez L, *et al.* Predictors of nonalcoholic steatohepatitis (NASH) in obese

patients undergoing gastric bypass. Obes Surg 2005; 15(8): 1148-53.
[http://dx.doi.org/10.1381/0960892055002347] [PMID: 16197788]

[32]   Haentjens P, Massaad D, Reynaert H, *et al.* Identifying non-alcoholic fatty liver disease among asymptomatic overweight and obese individuals by clinical and biochemical characteristics. Acta Clin Belg 2009; 64(6): 483-93.
[http://dx.doi.org/10.1179/acb.2009.084] [PMID: 20101871]

[33]   Wree A, Schlattjan M, Bechmann LP, *et al.* Adipocyte cell size, free fatty acids and apolipoproteins are associated with non-alcoholic liver injury progression in severely obese patients. Metabolism 2014; 63(12): 1542-52.
[http://dx.doi.org/10.1016/j.metabol.2014.09.001] [PMID: 25267016]

[34]   OConnell J, Lynch L, Cawood TJ, *et al.* The relationship of omental and subcutaneous adipocyte size to metabolic disease in severe obesity. PLoS One 2010; 5(4): e9997.
[http://dx.doi.org/10.1371/journal.pone.0009997] [PMID: 20376319]

[35]   Koppe SW. Obesity and the liver: nonalcoholic fatty liver disease. Transl Res 2014; 164(4): 312-22.
[http://dx.doi.org/10.1016/j.trsl.2014.06.008] [PMID: 25028077]

[36]   Promrat K, Kleiner DE, Niemeier HM, *et al.* Randomized controlled trial testing the effects of weight loss on nonalcoholic steatohepatitis. Hepatology 2010; 51(1): 121-9.
[http://dx.doi.org/10.1002/hep.23276] [PMID: 19827166]

[37]   Harrison SA, Fecht W, Brunt EM, Neuschwander-Tetri BA. Orlistat for overweight subjects with nonalcoholic steatohepatitis: A randomized, prospective trial. Hepatology 2009; 49(1): 80-6.
[http://dx.doi.org/10.1002/hep.22575] [PMID: 19053049]

[38]   Andersen T, Gluud C, Franzmann MB, Christoffersen P. Hepatic effects of dietary weight loss in morbidly obese subjects. J Hepatol 1991; 12(2): 224-9.
[http://dx.doi.org/10.1016/0168-8278(91)90942-5] [PMID: 2051001]

[39]   Whiting DR, Guariguata L, Weil C, Shaw J. IDF diabetes atlas: global estimates of the prevalence of diabetes for 2011 and 2030. Diabetes Res Clin Pract 2011; 94(3): 311-21.
[http://dx.doi.org/10.1016/j.diabres.2011.10.029] [PMID: 22079683]

[40]   Economic costs of diabetes in the U.S. In 2007. Diabetes Care 2008; 31(3): 596-615.
[http://dx.doi.org/10.2337/dc08-9017] [PMID: 18308683]

[41]   Pappachan JM, Antonio FA, Edavalath M, Mukherjee A. Non-alcoholic fatty liver disease: a diabetologists perspective. Endocrine 2014; 45(3): 344-53.
[http://dx.doi.org/10.1007/s12020-013-0087-8] [PMID: 24287794]

[42]   Williams KH, Shackel NA, Gorrell MD, McLennan SV, Twigg SM. Diabetes and nonalcoholic Fatty liver disease: a pathogenic duo. Endocr Rev 2013; 34(1): 84-129.
[http://dx.doi.org/10.1210/er.2012-1009] [PMID: 23238855]

[43]   Targher G, Bertolini L, Padovani R, *et al.* Increased prevalence of cardiovascular disease in Type 2 diabetic patients with non-alcoholic fatty liver disease. Diabet Med 2006; 23(4): 403-9.
[http://dx.doi.org/10.1111/j.1464-5491.2006.01817.x] [PMID: 16620269]

[44]   Catalano D, Trovato GM, Martines GF, Pirri C, Trovato FM. Renal function and severity of bright liver. Relationship with insulin resistance, intrarenal resistive index, and glomerular filtration rate. Hepatol Int 2011; 5(3): 822-9.
[http://dx.doi.org/10.1007/s12072-011-9254-2] [PMID: 21484130]

[45]   Targher G, Chonchol M, Zoppini G, Abaterusso C, Bonora E. Risk of chronic kidney disease in patients with non-alcoholic fatty liver disease: is there a link? J Hepatol 2011; 54(5): 1020-9.
[http://dx.doi.org/10.1016/j.jhep.2010.11.007] [PMID: 21145850]

[46]   Targher G, Bertolini L, Rodella S, Lippi G, Zoppini G, Chonchol M. Relationship between kidney

function and liver histology in subjects with nonalcoholic steatohepatitis. Clin J Am Soc Nephrol 2010; 5(12): 2166-71.
[http://dx.doi.org/10.2215/CJN.05050610] [PMID: 20724519]

[47] Lv WS, Sun RX, Gao YY, *et al.* Nonalcoholic fatty liver disease and microvascular complications in type 2 diabetes. World J Gastroenterol 2013; 19(20): 3134-42.
[http://dx.doi.org/10.3748/wjg.v19.i20.3134] [PMID: 23716995]

[48] Musso G, Cassader M, Gambino R. Cholesterol-lowering therapy for the treatment of nonalcoholic fatty liver disease: an update. Curr Opin Lipidol 2011; 22(6): 489-96.
[http://dx.doi.org/10.1097/MOL.0b013e32834c37ee] [PMID: 21986643]

[49] Manchanayake J, Chitturi S, Nolan C, Farrell GC. Postprandial hyperinsulinemia is universal in non-diabetic patients with nonalcoholic fatty liver disease. J Gastroenterol Hepatol 2011; 26(3): 510-6.
[http://dx.doi.org/10.1111/j.1440-1746.2010.06528.x] [PMID: 21155882]

[50] Kimura Y, Hyogo H, Ishitobi T, Nabeshima Y, Arihiro K, Chayama K. Postprandial insulin secretion pattern is associated with histological severity in non-alcoholic fatty liver disease patients without prior known diabetes mellitus. J Gastroenterol Hepatol 2011; 26(3): 517-22.
[http://dx.doi.org/10.1111/j.1440-1746.2010.06567.x] [PMID: 21054523]

[51] Ortiz-Lopez C, Lomonaco R, Orsak B, *et al.* Prevalence of prediabetes and diabetes and metabolic profile of patients with nonalcoholic fatty liver disease (NAFLD). Diabetes Care 2012; 35(4): 873-8.
[http://dx.doi.org/10.2337/dc11-1849] [PMID: 22374640]

[52] Hossain N, Afendy A, Stepanova M, *et al.* Independent predictors of fibrosis in patients with nonalcoholic fatty liver disease. Clin Gastroenterol Hepatol 2009; 7(11): 1224-1229, 1229.e1-1229.e2.
[http://dx.doi.org/10.1016/j.cgh.2009.06.007] [PMID: 19559819]

[53] Beymer C, Kowdley KV, Larson A, Edmonson P, Dellinger EP, Flum DR. Prevalence and predictors of asymptomatic liver disease in patients undergoing gastric bypass surgery. Arch Surg 2003; 138(11): 1240-4.
[http://dx.doi.org/10.1001/archsurg.138.11.1240] [PMID: 14609874]

[54] Uygun A, Kadayifci A, Isik AT, *et al.* Metformin in the treatment of patients with non-alcoholic steatohepatitis. Aliment Pharmacol Ther 2004; 19(5): 537-44.
[http://dx.doi.org/10.1111/j.1365-2036.2004.01888.x] [PMID: 14987322]

[55] Bugianesi E, Gentilcore E, Manini R, *et al.* A randomized controlled trial of metformin *versus* vitamin E or prescriptive diet in nonalcoholic fatty liver disease. Am J Gastroenterol 2005; 100(5): 1082-90.
[http://dx.doi.org/10.1111/j.1572-0241.2005.41583.x] [PMID: 15842582]

[56] Aithal GP, Thomas JA, Kaye PV, *et al.* Randomized, placebo-controlled trial of pioglitazone in nondiabetic subjects with nonalcoholic steatohepatitis. Gastroenterology 2008; 135(4): 1176-84.
[http://dx.doi.org/10.1053/j.gastro.2008.06.047] [PMID: 18718471]

[57] Sanyal AJ, Chalasani N, Kowdley KV, *et al.* Pioglitazone, vitamin E, or placebo for nonalcoholic steatohepatitis. N Engl J Med 2010; 362(18): 1675-85.
[http://dx.doi.org/10.1056/NEJMoa0907929] [PMID: 20427778]

[58] Mendoza C, Ali R, Mathew M, Chen J, Diaz N, Kaminski-Graham R. Exenatide promotes weight loss and improves insulin secretion, subclinical inflammation, and hepatic steatosis when replaced for pre-meal insulin in T2DM patients. Diabetes 2009; 58 (Suppl. 1): A507.

[59] Kenny PR, Brady DE, Torres DM, Ragozzino L, Chalasani N, Harrison SA. Exenatide in the treatment of diabetic patients with non-alcoholic steatohepatitis: a case series. Am J Gastroenterol 2010; 105(12): 2707-9.
[http://dx.doi.org/10.1038/ajg.2010.363] [PMID: 21131943]

[60] Balaban YH, Korkusuz P, Simsek H, *et al.* Dipeptidyl peptidase IV (DDP IV) in NASH patients. Ann

Hepatol 2007; 6(4): 242-50.
[PMID: 18007554]

[61]   Schuppan D, Schattenberg JM. Non-alcoholic steatohepatitis: pathogenesis and novel therapeutic approaches. J Gastroenterol Hepatol 2013; 28 (Suppl. 1): 68-76.
[http://dx.doi.org/10.1111/jgh.12212] [PMID: 23855299]

[62]   Ábel T. The new therapy of type 2 diabetes: DDP-4 inhibitors. Hypoglycemia INTECH. 2011; pp. 1-14.

[63]   Wierzbicki AS, Oben J. Nonalcoholic fatty liver disease and lipids. Curr Opin Lipidol 2012; 23(4): 345-52.
[http://dx.doi.org/10.1097/MOL.0b013e3283541cfc] [PMID: 22617751]

[64]   Kim HJ, Kim HJ, Lee KE, *et al.* Metabolic significance of nonalcoholic fatty liver disease in nonobese, nondiabetic adults. Arch Intern Med 2004; 164(19): 2169-75.
[http://dx.doi.org/10.1001/archinte.164.19.2169] [PMID: 15505132]

[65]   Toledo FG, Sniderman AD, Kelley DE. Influence of hepatic steatosis (fatty liver) on severity and composition of dyslipidemia in type 2 diabetes. Diabetes Care 2006; 29(8): 1845-50.
[http://dx.doi.org/10.2337/dc06-0455] [PMID: 16873790]

[66]   DeFilippis AP, Blaha MJ, Martin SS, *et al.* Nonalcoholic fatty liver disease and serum lipoproteins: the Multi-Ethnic Study of Atherosclerosis. Atherosclerosis 2013; 227(2): 429-36.
[http://dx.doi.org/10.1016/j.atherosclerosis.2013.01.022] [PMID: 23419204]

[67]   Adiels M, Taskinen MR, Borén J. Fatty liver, insulin resistance, and dyslipidemia. Curr Diab Rep 2008; 8(1): 60-4.
[http://dx.doi.org/10.1007/s11892-008-0011-4] [PMID: 18367000]

[68]   Sniderman A, Couture P, de Graaf J. Diagnosis and treatment of apolipoprotein B dyslipoproteinemias. Nat Rev Endocrinol 2010; 6(6): 335-46.
[http://dx.doi.org/10.1038/nrendo.2010.50] [PMID: 20421882]

[69]   Ridker PM, Cook NR. Statins: new American guidelines for prevention of cardiovascular disease. Lancet 2013; 382(9907): 1762-5.
[http://dx.doi.org/10.1016/S0140-6736(13)62388-0] [PMID: 24268611]

[70]   Younossi ZM, Reyes MJ, Mishra A, Mehta R, Henry L. Systematic review with meta-analysis: non-alcoholic steatohepatitis - a case for personalised treatment based on pathogenic targets. Aliment Pharmacol Ther 2014; 39(1): 3-14.
[http://dx.doi.org/10.1111/apt.12543] [PMID: 24206433]

[71]   Halcox JP, Deanfield JE. Beyond the laboratory: clinical implications for statin pleiotropy. Circulation 2004; 109((21 Suppl 1)): 42-8.
[http://dx.doi.org/10.1161/01.CIR.0000129500.29229.92]

[72]   Kiyici M, Gulten M, Gurel S, *et al.* Ursodeoxycholic acid and atorvastatin in the treatment of nonalcoholic steatohepatitis. Can J Gastroenterol 2003; 17(12): 713-8.
[http://dx.doi.org/10.1155/2003/857869] [PMID: 14679419]

[73]   Hatzitolios A, Savopoulos C, Lazaraki G, *et al.* Efficacy of omega-3 fatty acids, atorvastatin and orlistat in non-alcoholic fatty liver disease with dyslipidemia. Indian J Gastroenterol 2004; 23(4): 131-4.
[PMID: 15333967]

[74]   Gómez-Domínguez E, Gisbert JP, Moreno-Monteagudo JA, García-Buey L, Moreno-Otero R. A pilot study of atorvastatin treatment in dyslipemid, non-alcoholic fatty liver patients. Aliment Pharmacol Ther 2006; 23(11): 1643-7.
[http://dx.doi.org/10.1111/j.1365-2036.2006.02926.x] [PMID: 16696815]

[75]   Kimura Y, Hyogo H, Yamagishi S, *et al.* Atorvastatin decreases serum levels of advanced glycation endproducts (AGEs) in nonalcoholic steatohepatitis (NASH) patients with dyslipidemia: clinical usefulness of AGEs as a biomarker for the attenuation of NASH. J Gastroenterol 2010; 45(7): 750-7.
[http://dx.doi.org/10.1007/s00535-010-0203-y] [PMID: 20112031]

[76]   Chalasani N, Younossi Z, Lavine JE, *et al.* The diagnosis and management of non-alcoholic fatty liver disease: practice Guideline by the American Association for the Study of Liver Diseases, American College of Gastroenterology, and the American Gastroenterological Association. Hepatology 2012; 55(6): 2005-23.
[http://dx.doi.org/10.1002/hep.25762] [PMID: 22488764]

[77]   Yoneda M, Fujita K, Nozaki Y, *et al.* Efficacy of ezetimibe for the treatment of nonalcoholic steatohepatitis: an open label, pilot study. Hepatol Res 2010; 40: 613-21.
[http://dx.doi.org/10.1111/j.1872-034X.2010.00644.x] [PMID: 20412328]

[78]   Park H, Shima T, Yamaguchi K, *et al.* Efficacy of long-term ezetimibe therapy in patients with nonalcoholic fatty liver disease. J Gastroenterol 2011; 46(1): 101-7.
[http://dx.doi.org/10.1007/s00535-010-0291-8] [PMID: 20658156]

[79]   Ábel T, Fehér J, Dinya E, Eldin MG, Kovács A. Safety and efficacy of combined ezetimibe/simvastatin treatment and simvastatin monotherapy in patients with non-alcoholic fatty liver disease. Med Sci Monit 2009; 15(12): MS6-MS11.
[PMID: 19946244]

[80]   Athyros VG, Mikhailidis DP, Didangelos TP, *et al.* Effect of multifactorial treatment on non-alcoholic fatty liver disease in metabolic syndrome: a randomised study. Curr Med Res Opin 2006; 22(5): 873-83.
[http://dx.doi.org/10.1185/030079906X104696] [PMID: 16709309]

[81]   Fernández-Miranda C, Pérez-Carreras M, Colina F, López-Alonso G, Vargas C, Solís-Herruzo JA. A pilot trial of fenofibrate for the treatment of non-alcoholic fatty liver disease. Dig Liver Dis 2008; 40(3): 200-5.
[http://dx.doi.org/10.1016/j.dld.2007.10.002] [PMID: 18261709]

[82]   Fabbrini E, Mohammed BS, Korenblat KM, *et al.* Effect of fenofibrate and niacin on intrahepatic triglyceride content, very low-density lipoprotein kinetics, and insulin action in obese subjects with nonalcoholic fatty liver disease. J Clin Endocrinol Metab 2010; 95(6): 2727-35.
[http://dx.doi.org/10.1210/jc.2009-2622] [PMID: 20371660]

[83]   Belfort R, Berria R, Cornell J, Cusi K. Fenofibrate reduces systemic inflammation markers independent of its effects on lipid and glucose metabolism in patients with the metabolic syndrome. J Clin Endocrinol Metab 2010; 95(2): 829-36.
[http://dx.doi.org/10.1210/jc.2009-1487] [PMID: 20061429]

[84]   López-Suárez A, Guerrero JM, Elvira-González J, Beltrán-Robles M, Cañas-Hormigo F, Bascuñana-Quirell A. Nonalcoholic fatty liver disease is associated with blood pressure in hypertensive and nonhypertensive individuals from the general population with normal levels of alanine aminotransferase. Eur J Gastroenterol Hepatol 2011; 23(11): 1011-7.

[85]   Fallo F, Dalla Pozza A, Sonino N, *et al.* Nonalcoholic fatty liver disease, adiponectin and insulin resistance in dipper and nondipper essential hypertensive patients. J Hypertens 2008; 26(11): 2191-7.
[http://dx.doi.org/10.1097/HJH.0b013e32830dfe4b] [PMID: 18854760]

[86]   Lau K, Lorbeer R, Haring R, *et al.* The association between fatty liver disease and blood pressure in a population-based prospective longitudinal study. J Hypertens 2010; 28(9): 1829-35.
[http://dx.doi.org/10.1097/HJH.0b013e32833c211b] [PMID: 20577126]

[87]   Fallo F, Dalla Pozza A, Sonino N, *et al.* Non-alcoholic fatty liver disease is associated with left ventricular diastolic dysfunction in essential hypertension. Nutr Metab Cardiovasc Dis 2009; 19(9):

646-53.
[http://dx.doi.org/10.1016/j.numecd.2008.12.007] [PMID: 19278843]

[88] Mantovani A, Zoppini G, Targher G, Golia G, Bonora E. Non-alcoholic fatty liver disease is independently associated with left ventricular hypertrophy in hypertensive Type 2 diabetic individuals. J Endocrinol Invest 2012; 35(2): 215-8.
[http://dx.doi.org/10.1007/BF03345421] [PMID: 22490991]

[89] Liu YC, Hung CS, Wu YW, *et al.* Influence of non-alcoholic fatty liver disease on autonomic changes evaluated by the time domain, frequency domain, and symbolic dynamics of heart rate variability. PLoS One 2013; 8(4): e61803.
[http://dx.doi.org/10.1371/journal.pone.0061803] [PMID: 23626730]

[90] Dixon JB, Bhathal PS, OBrien PE. Nonalcoholic fatty liver disease: predictors of nonalcoholic steatohepatitis and liver fibrosis in the severely obese. Gastroenterology 2001; 121(1): 91-100.
[http://dx.doi.org/10.1053/gast.2001.25540] [PMID: 11438497]

[91] Angulo P. Nonalcoholic fatty liver disease. N Engl J Med 2002; 346(16): 1221-31.
[http://dx.doi.org/10.1056/NEJMra011775] [PMID: 11961152]

[92] Chalasani N, Younossi Z, Lavine JE, *et al.* The diagnosis and management of non-alcoholic fatty liver disease: practice Guideline by the American Association for the Study of Liver Diseases, American College of Gastroenterology, and the American Gastroenterological Association. Hepatology 2012; 55(6): 2005-23.
[http://dx.doi.org/10.1002/hep.25762] [PMID: 22488764]

[93] Donati G, Stagni B, Piscaglia F, *et al.* Increased prevalence of fatty liver in arterial hypertensive patients with normal liver enzymes: role of insulin resistance. Gut 2004; 53(7): 1020-3.
[http://dx.doi.org/10.1136/gut.2003.027086] [PMID: 15194655]

[94] Younossi ZM, Stepanova M, Negro F, *et al.* Nonalcoholic fatty liver disease in lean individuals in the United States. Medicine (Baltimore) 2012; 91(6): 319-27.
[http://dx.doi.org/10.1097/MD.0b013e3182779d49] [PMID: 23117851]

[95] Aneni EC, Oni ET, Martin SS, *et al.* Blood pressure is associated with the presence and severity of nonalcoholic fatty liver disease across the spectrum of cardiometabolic risk. J Hypertens 2015; 33(6): 1207-14.
[http://dx.doi.org/10.1097/HJH.0000000000000532] [PMID: 25693058]

[96] Chitturi S, Abeygunasekera S, Farrell GC, *et al.* NASH and insulin resistance: Insulin hypersecretion and specific association with the insulin resistance syndrome. Hepatology 2002; 35(2): 373-9.
[http://dx.doi.org/10.1053/jhep.2002.30692] [PMID: 11826411]

[97] Cusi K. Nonalcoholic fatty liver disease in type 2 diabetes mellitus. Curr Opin Endocrinol Diabetes Obes 2009; 16(2): 141-9.
[http://dx.doi.org/10.1097/MED.0b013e3283293015] [PMID: 19262374]

[98] Fabbrini E, Sullivan S, Klein S. Obesity and nonalcoholic fatty liver disease: biochemical, metabolic, and clinical implications. Hepatology 2010; 51(2): 679-89.
[http://dx.doi.org/10.1002/hep.23280] [PMID: 20041406]

[99] Alberti KG, Zimmet P, Shaw J. The metabolic syndromea new worldwide definition. Lancet 2005; 366(9491): 1059-62.
[http://dx.doi.org/10.1016/S0140-6736(05)67402-8] [PMID: 16182882]

[100] Marceau P, Biron S, Hould FS, *et al.* Liver pathology and the metabolic syndrome X in severe obesity. J Clin Endocrinol Metab 1999; 84(5): 1513-7.
[http://dx.doi.org/10.1210/jcem.84.5.5661] [PMID: 10323371]

[101]   Lonardo A, Ballestri S, Marchesini G, Angulo P, Loria P. Nonalcoholic fatty liver disease: a precursor of the metabolic syndrome. Dig Liver Dis 2015; 47(3): 181-90.
[http://dx.doi.org/10.1016/j.dld.2014.09.020] [PMID: 25739820]

CHAPTER 7

Management of NAFLD

Krisztina Hagymási[*] and **Gabriella Lengyel**

Semmelweis University, 2ⁿᵈ Department of Internal Medicine, Budapest, Hungary

Abstract: Nonalcoholic fatty liver disease and steatohepatitis are the most common chronic diseases of the liver. The process of their development has not yet been fully elucidated. It is characterized by insulin resistance, hepatic lipid accumulation with a secondary pathologic production of free radicals that induce inflammatory processes and fibrosis. There is no evidence-based therapy. It is important to eliminate the pathogenic factors (excess body weight, disordered carbohydrate metabolism, and hyperlipidemia). Potential modalities of a causal therapy include cannabinoid receptor 1 antagonists which do not cross the blood-brain barrier, cannabinoid receptor 2 agonists; selective serotonin 2C receptor agonist, thiazolidinediones, incretins, and dipeptidyl peptidase inhibitors. Additional therapeutic possibilities of the future may target antioxidant defense, immune-mediated mechanisms, apoptosis, and lipogenesis.

Keywords: Diabetes mellitus, Dipeptidyl peptidase inhibitors, Hyperlipidemia, Incretins, Insulin resistance, Lifestyle modification, Nonalcoholic steatohepatitis, Nonalcoholic steatosis, Thiazolidinediones, Treatment, Vitamin E, Weight loss.

INTRODUCTION

Nonalcoholic fatty liver disease (NAFLD) is an acquired hepatic disease that may be characterized, in addition to lipid accumulation, by lobular inflammation (nonalcoholic steatohepatitis, NASH), accruement of connective tissue (fibrosis) and fibrotic remodeling (cirrhosis) [1].

NAFLD is the most frequent chronic liver disease, which is the most common cause of hepatic dysfunction [2]. Depending on the method of screening, NAFLD may affect 20% population on average (6 to 33%), however, according to more recent data 30 to 50% of the population [1 - 6]. Its prevalence is increasing all over the world, unfortunately also among children [1, 7] due to the epidemic spread of obesity [1]. The long-term prognosis of NAFLD is good. The associated

[*] **Corresponding author Krisztina Hagymási:** Semmelweis University, 2ⁿᵈ Department of Internal Medicine, Budapest, Hungary; Tel: (+36-1)266 09 01/ Fax: (+36-1)266 08 16; E-mail: hagymasi.krisztina@med.semmelweis-univ.hu

Tatjana Ábel & Gabriella Lengyel (Eds.)
All rights reserved-© 2017 Bentham Science Publishers

mortality is similar to that of the general population; however, it is also influenced by the accompanying diseases. The liver mortality of NASH is three times higher in comparison to the simple hepatic steatosis (8.6% *vs.* 1.7%) [1]. Its importance is further increased by the fact that it is a pathogenic factor of hepatocellular carcinoma [3, 8]. In patients with chronic HCV infection the prevalence of steatosis has been estimated to be about 55% [9, 10]. The viral steatosis (genotype 3) and metabolic (non-3 genotype) steatosis predict a more rapid progression of fibrosis, an increased risk of development of hepatocellular carcinoma, and a negative response rate to interferon-based treatment [9].

NAFLD may occur in patients of all ages, with an average of 47 to 53 years [2]. Its prevalence increases with the age; it is determined by genetic and environmental factors [1]. As for the involvement of genders, data of literature are equivocal. Certainly, the course of the disease is different in male and female patients [6]. Patients (69 to 100%) are obese (BMI >30 kg/m^2); they often have type 2 diabetes mellitus (34 to 75%) or hyperlipidemia (20 to 81%), and almost a half of them have hypertension [2].

The development of NAFLD and the process of its progression have not yet been fully elucidated. Its pathogenetic mechanism is characterized by the theory of 'double hits': 1) accumulation of triglycerides in the liver, and then 2) pathologic production of free radicals inducing inflammatory processes and fibrosis formation [2]. Increased uptake of fatty acids by the hepatocytes, decreased uptake of lipoproteins by the tissues, increased *de novo* hepatic lipogenesis, decreased hepatic output of triglycerides and decreased mitochondrial fatty acid oxidation may all contribute to hepatic steatosis [2, 11]. The development of *insulin resistance* is a key event in the development of fatty liver [11 - 15].

The accruement of fatty acids induces a secondary *release of free radicals* by activating the microsomal monooxygenase system, as well as by mitochondrial β-oxidation and peroxisomal ω-oxidation of the free fatty acids, which results in lipid peroxidation and a damage of proteins and DNA. Products of lipid peroxidation inhibit the delivery of triglycerides from the liver, thus making the steatosis more severe. Increased expression of tumor necrosis factor alpha (TNF-α) and transforming growth factor beta (TGF-β) lead to necrosis of hepatocytes and inflammation; these molecular events promote the transformation of stellate cells to collagen-producing myofibroblasts and the fibrogenesis. Free radical processes are also enhanced by portal endotoxemia, mitochondrial disorders, leptin production of the stellate cells, and moderate accruement of iron [12, 13, 16, 17] (Fig. **1**).

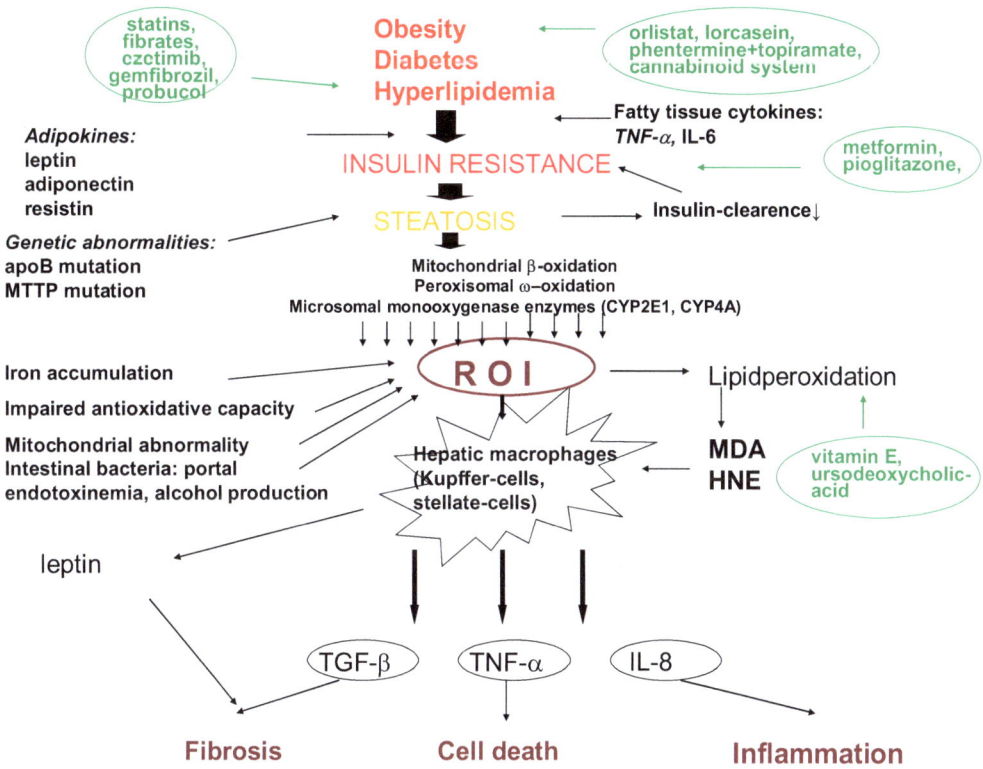

Fig. (1). Pathogenesis of NAFLD and NASH, and the possibilities of the therapy.

HNE=hydroxynonenal; IL-8= interleukin-8; MDA= malondialdehyde; MTTP= microsomal triglyceride transfer protein; ROI= reactive oxygen species; TGF-β= transforming growth factor-β; TNF-α=tumor necrosis factor-α

There is no known, evidence-based specific therapy. The management of patients with NAFLD includes treating of metabolic co-morbidities, such as obesity, hyperlipidemia, insulin resistance, and diabetes mellitus [3]. A second strategy is to prevent/reverse hepatic cellular damage induced by lipotoxicity. This can be achieved by inhibiting lipid peroxidation and oxidative stress, or through the use of anti-inflammatory, anti-apoptotic or other hepatoprotective agents. These two strategies may be combined at best [17 - 21].

Treatment

Reduction of Body Weight

Gradual reduction of body weight, together with concomitant use of diet and physical activity, improves insulin sensitivity and mitigates the histological abnormities [22]. Baseline body weight should be reduced by 5 to 10%, with a 0.45 to 0.9 kg per week rate of decrease. Rapid weight loss is unfavorable, as it increases portal inflammation and fibrosis [4]. A reduction of body weight by 7 to 10% may moderate hepatic steatosis by 42 to 51%, while a reduction at 5% or below has no considerable impact on the hepatic lipid content [1].

Diet

There are no exact recommendations for a composition of the diet [1, 23, 24]. The consumption of saturated fats, sugary drinks, or food with a high glycemic index should be avoided [25]. Ingestion of *fructose* is an independent factor of the development of NAFLD and metabolic syndrome. Unlike glucose, fructose does not stimulate leptin secretion and causes no satiety, at the same time it stimulates *de novo* lipogenesis. Therefore, the consumption of fructose-containing food and drinks should be avoided [26]. However, *Johnston et al.* indicated an energy-mediated, rather than a specific macronutrient-mediated, effect. In the isocaloric period, overweight men who were on a high-fructose or a high-glucose diet did not develop any significant changes in hepatic triacylglycerol concentration or serum levels of liver enzymes. However, in the hypercaloric period, both high-fructose and high-glucose diets produced significant increases in these parameters without any significant difference between the 2 groups [27]. The *n-3/n-6 polyunsaturated fatty acids* decrease triglyceride levels and the size of intramuscular lipid drops; they have been shown to improve insulin resistance and enhance non-hepatic glucose utilization [28]. *Omega-3 fatty acids* may exert a beneficial influence on the hepatic lipid metabolism, on adipose tissue function and on the inflammation. By binding to the peroxisome proliferator activated receptor alpha (PPARα) and activating it, omega-3 fatty acids stimulate lipid oxidation, and by inhibiting the expression of the sterol regulatory element binding protein-1c (SREBP-1c) gene they inhibit lipogenesis [29]. Further studies are required in relation to the exact dosage and the effects on the various components of NAFLD (steatosis, inflammation, fibrosis) [30].

Coffee consumption reduces the risk of NAFLD, the extent of hepatic steatosis, as well as the risk of fibrosis in patients with NASH. Coffee contains more than 1000 compounds. Its main components include caffeine, diterpenes as cafestol and kahweol, as well as chlorogenic acid. Underlying its beneficial effects, there may be its antioxidant (stimulation of antioxidant responsive element-regulated signal transduction), antifibrotic (down-regulation of TGF-β-induced connective tissue growth factor production, inhibition of focal adhesion kinase and actin synthesis, stimulation of hepatic stellate cell apoptosis and expression of intracellular F-actin and cAMP, inhibition of expression of procollagen type 1C and alpha-smooth muscle actin expression) effects [31].

It is generally recommended that patients with NAFLD should not consume alcohol. Non-heavy alcohol consumption may have paradoxical and favorable hepatic effects, presumably due to its effects on insulin sensitivity and other metabolic parameters. Light and moderate alcohol consumption is inversely associated with prevalence of fatty liver, and is associated with favorable hepatic histology [32]. Some components of wine, aside from alcohol, such as natural polyphenols may be playing a role in this phenomenon. In a mouse model of fatty liver, natural polyphenol resveratrol improved insulin resistance and reduced the development of fatty liver, which may be in relation to the inhibition of sterol regulatory element-binding protein-1c, a key transcription factor in lipogenesis, reducing oxidative damage, and amelioration of lipid peroxidation [32, 33]. Until further data from rigorous prospective studies become available, people with NAFLD should avoid alcohol of any type or amount [32].

Physical Activity

Physical activity decreases insulin resistance (by enhancing the expression of glucose transporter-4) and it exerts a beneficial effect on the hepatic lipid content. Moderate to high physical activity for 30 minutes on 3 to 5 occasions per week is recommended [1].

Pharmacotherapy

Pharmacological treatment of obesity may be offered in patients with a body mass index (BMI) >30 kg/m^2, or in overweight patients (BMI=27.0-29.9 kg/m^2) with obesity related comorbidities [34]. The marketing authorizations of *sibutramine,* that inhibits monoamine reuptake and in this way increases postprandial satiety, reduces food intake and enhances the effluence of energy, have been suspended by the European Medicines Agency [35]. *Orlistat* creates a covalent bond with the lipases in the gastrointestinal system and neutralizes the enzyme, so that it is unable to cleave the fat content of the food, which is in the form of triglyceride, into absorbable free fatty acids and monoglycerides. The effects of orlistat on histological abnormities of the liver in NAFLD are equivocal [1].

The selective cannabinoid receptor-1 antagonist, *rimonabant* that reduces food and energy intake and thus body weight, and reverses hepatic steatosis, as well as improves insulin sensitivity, was also withdrawn from the market due to its side effects causing mood disorders. The use of *cannabinoid receptor-1 (CB1R) antagonists* which do not cross the blood-brain barrier (AM 6545, JD 5037) still requires confirmation [36 - 38] in clinical models [38]. Preliminary results indicate that AM6545 displays antifibrogenic effects similar to rimonabant [36]. The peripherally restricted CB1R antagonist JD5037 is equieffective with its brain-penetrant parent compound in reducing appetite, body weight, hepatic steatosis, and insulin resistance [39]. Cannabinoid receptors-2 (CB2R) predominantly displays protective properties during liver injury *via* anti-inflammatory and antifibrogenic signals [36, 37]. They have no impact on either food intake or body weight progression. CB2 agonists may also offer a promising modality; their testing is currently in a preclinical stage [36, 37].

The selective serotonin-2C receptor agonist, *lorcaserin* causes satiety and reduces the appetite; similarly, the combination of the noradrenergic sympathomimetic *phentermine* and the antiepileptic *topiramate* (phentermine-topiramate) has been approved by the Food and Drug Administration as medicines for reducing the body weight. Although the experience with their use in patients with NAFLD is still lacking, they may offer promising modalities [40].

Surgical solutions (laparoscopic Roux-en-Y gastric bypass, laparoscopic adjustable gastric banding, laparoscopic sleeve gastrectomy) may be considered for body weight reduction in severely obese patients (BMI >35 kg/m^2 + cardiovascular complications, or BMI >40 kg/m^2) [41]. Based on the results of a metaanalysis, bariatric surgical procedures reduced steatosis, histological abnormities of NASH, and hepatic fibrosis in 92%, 81% and 66% of patients, respectively [42]. At the same time, their effect on the accumulation of connective tissue is equivocal; increasing fibrosis has also been reported [43]. Due to an excessive reduction of the body weight, fulminant steatohepatitis also developed in rare cases during the first postoperative year [26].

Improving Insulin Sensitivity

Metformin improves insulin sensitivity by reducing hepatic glucose production and stimulating the uptake of glucose by skeletal muscles. It reduces hepatic TNF-α expression, stimulates fatty acid oxidation, and inhibits lipogenesis [2]. It improves the abnormities of hepatic enzymes; while its effects on steatosis, inflammation and fibrosis are equivocal. The American Gastroenterological Association (AGA), the American Association for the Study of Liver Diseases (AASLD) and the American College of Gastroenterology (ACG) do not recommend its use [3].

Thiazolidinediones are insulin sensitizers which act through the peroxisome prolifcrator activated receptor-γ. Through its pleiotropic effects, *pioglitazone* improves endothelial dysfunction, reduces blood pressure, improves diabetic dyslipidemia, and decreases the levels of circulating inflammatory cytokines and prothrombotic factors [44]. It moderates the activity of transaminases, as well as steatosis, inflammation and ballooning degeneration. Its effect on fibrosis is ambiguous [26]. The use of *pioglitazone* is recommended in patients with histologically confirmed NASH; however, long-term studies are required in order to exactly assess the efficacy and safety of the medicine [3].

Glucagon-like peptide 1 (GLP-1), an *incretin* originating from the gastrointestinal tract, plays a role in the regulation of energy balance and food intake. It stimulates glucose-dependent insulin secretion, inhibits glucagon secretion, delays gastric emptying, and reduces the appetite [45]. Agonists of its receptor (GLP-1-RA) enhance insulin secretion and inhibit glucagon secretion. Studies with GLP-1 receptor antagonists (*exenatide*) or inhibitors of the enzyme degrading GLP-1 (dipeptidyl peptidase-IV, DPP-IV) (*sitagliptin*) are in progress in patients with type 2 diabetes mellitus. *Exenatide* (*exendin-4*), a GLP-1-RA with a longer half-life due to its resistance to DPP-IV, reversed hepatic steatosis in *in vitro* studies in human hepatocyte cell lines [46] and in animal experiments [24, 46]. In human studies *exenatide* mitigated transaminase activity and reduced hepatic steatosis, as confirmed by proton magnetic resonance spectroscopy (1H-MRS) in a case report and in a study with a low number of cases [45, 47]. Its effect on the hepatic lesion was assessed without a histological confirmation [45, 48 - 50]. The DPP-IV inhibitor *sitagliptin* reduced transaminase activity [51, 52]; histological examinations revealed a marginally significant reduction in relation to balloon formation, NASH score and steatosis [52].

Liraglutide, a GLP-1-RA with a longer half-life, reduced transaminase activity in patients with type 2 diabetes mellitus [53, 54]. The control of diabetes mellitus also markedly improved, whereas fast blood glucose and HbA1c decreased. Additionally, there was a significant improvement of liver fibrosis score (APRI index) [53]. It was safe and well-tolerated [53, 54].

The short-acting insulin secretagogue *repaglinide* and *nateglinide* may be potential therapeutic modalities for NAFLD. In patients with type 2 diabetes mellitus, nateglinide improved carbohydrate balance, reduced hepatic enzyme abnormities as well as the histological abnormities of NAFLD [55].

Reduction of Lipid Levels

Based on the currently available data, no major risk of hepatic impairment is to be reckoned with when using the HMG-CoA reductase inhibitor statins. They reduce transaminase activity; however, it is not clear whether it is due to statin therapy or to body weight reduction [1], and they also improve liver histology [3]. They are recommended by AGA, AASLD and ACG for treating lipid abnormalities in patients with NALD/NASH, with significant improvement of cardiovascular outcomes in patients with elevated liver enzymes, likely due to NAFLD. There are no randomized control trials with histological endpoints which investigated statins to treat NASH, for this reason statins should not be used to specifically treat NASH [3]. *Simvastatin* and *atorvastatin* are effective and safe. Further studies are needed to evaluate the efficacy and safety of *lovastatin, pravastatin, pitavastatin* and *rosuvastatin* [56].

Their antiphlogistic, antioxidant, antithrombotic, immunomodulating and antibacterial properties may also underlay the reduction of hepatic impairment [1].

Completion of statin therapy with *fibrates* has also been established in patients with high triglyceride and low HDL-cholesterol levels [57]. They are safe, they reduce hepatic enzyme abnormities, but they do not lead to a relevant reduction of the lipid content of the liver [1]. Administration of *gemfibrozil* for 4 weeks resulted in an improvement of hepatic function parameters (ALT, AST, GGT) in small-size prospective study. However, its effect on the histological abnormities was not studied [58].

Ezetimibe reduces intestinal cholesterol absorption by inhibiting the Niemann-Pick C1-Like 1 (NPC1L1) transporter. In studies with a low number of cases, it improved hepatic enzyme alterations and the abnormities of histology (except fibrosis), and it increased insulin sensitivity [59, 60].

Probucol, which also possesses an antioxidant effect, reduces cholesterol levels through a loss of bile acid-bound LDL-cholesterol with the feces, reduction of cholesterol synthesis and inhibition of enteral absorption; also decreased the activity of aminotransferases as well as steatosis and necro-inflammation; it exerted no effect on fibrosis [61].

Antioxidants

The lipophilic *Vitamin E*, which possesses antioxidant and antifibrotic activities, inhibits the expression of TNF-α and interleukins -1, -6 and -8 in monocytes and Kupffer cells. It hinders hepatic collagen α-1 gene expression and reduces the activity of transaminases. Its mitigating effect on the histological abnormities is equivocal. It reduces steatosis, inflammation and balloon formation, and it exerts no effect on fibrosis [26]. Undesirable effects have also been reported, supplementation of 400 IU per day increased all-cause mortality and the risk of prostate cancer as well [62, 63]. It is safe in patients with NASH who do not have type 2 diabetes mellitus. More long-term studies are needed in patients with type 2 diabetes mellitus and in those with NASH-cirrhosis, cryptogenic cirrhosis, and NAFLD without biopsy [3, 4]. It is recommended by AGA, AASLD and ACG in non-diabetic patients with histologically confirmed NASH [3].

Ursodeoxycholic Acid

Ursodeoxycholic acid (UDCA) inhibits apoptosis, arrests cellular regeneration, and blocks DNA repair. The anti-apoptosis is mediated *via* silencing of p53, inhibition of cyclin D1, and through caspase independent mechanism. UDCA inhibits co-enzyme A dependent steps in the cholesterol degradation, and conjugation of bile acids. It also inhibits degradation of nuclear factor kappaB (NF-kappaB) and its inhibitor kappaB, interacts with nuclear receptors that regulate gene-expression. UDCA is a steroid with immunomodulatory properties, suppresses interleukin-2, interleukin-4, and interferon-gamma, as well as IgM, IgG and IgA production. UDCA interferes with drug metabolism and detoxification as well [64].

UDCA reduces hepatic enzyme abnormities and improves carbohydrate metabolism and insulin sensitivity [65]. Its effect on the histological abnormities has not been demonstrated. Therefore, there is insufficient evidence supporting or refuting UDCA treatment of patients with NASH [4]. Its use is not recommended by AGA, AASLD and ACG [6].

Liver Transplantation

Liver transplantation for NASH was rarely performed until the beginning of the 1990s. Currently, it is the third most frequent cause for a liver transplantation [66]. Supposedly, cryptogenic cirrhosis due to NASH will be the leading indication of liver transplantation in 2020 [67]. 1-, 2-, and 3-year survival of patients who received a liver transplant because of NASH has been found to be excellent as 87.6%, 82.2% and 76.7%, respectively [68].

However, steatohepatitis often develops again in patients who underwent liver transplantation. The administered immunosuppressive therapy enhances the metabolic syndrome [66]. Post-transplant metabolic syndrome in recipients is at least twice as frequent in comparison to the general population [69], so fatty liver develops again, more commonly than in other conditions, and fibrosis may also develop very quickly in some cases [70, 71].

CONCLUDING REMARKS

The treatment of NAFLD is based on a changed lifestyle of the patients that is difficult to attain and to maintain. In addition to the changing lifestyle, the medication is individualized; it is determined by the associated diseases. Currently, thiazolidinediones and Vitamin E are the most promising therapeutic possibilities.

The occurring processes are not known in every detail, thus the therapeutic possibilities are controversial. Several questions are yet to be answered. It is not known whether hepatic steatosis is a cause or a consequence of the change of insulin sensitivity. A more exact knowledge on the pathogenesis of the disease may offer a more effective and safer therapeutic potential in the future.

Future therapeutic possibilities include: *anti-TNF-α antibodies (infliximab, adalimumab); pentoxifylline* that inhibits TNF-α production; the plasma membrane protein *caveolins*; the *IL-6 receptor antibody (tocilizumab); β-D-fructose* that decreases *de novo* hepatic lipogenesis; the angiotensin II receptor antagonist *losartan, telmisartan*; *acylation stimulating protein agonists*; the β.glucosidase inhibitor *acarbose*; *caspase inhibitors*; *liver-specific thyromimetics*; AMP-activated protein kinase activators (*oltipraz*); farnesoid X receptor agonists (*obeticholic acid*); as well as *pregnane X receptor agonists*; the antioxidant insulin-sensitizer *resveratrol*; the antioxidant *cysteamine bitartrate*; the selective type III phosphodiesterase inhibitor *cilostazol* which inhibits SREBP-1c expression, the synthetic retinoid *fenretinide*; the non-absorbable antibiotic *rifaximin* and the *probiotics* which exert their *effects on the intestinal flora* [1, 4, 16, 17, 72 - 75]. Table **1** summarizes the results of currently available human studies.

Table 1. List of drugs with a potential use in the therapy of NAFLD based on human studies.

	Effect	Ref	n	LF	S	I	F	Comment
Adalimumab	anti-TNF-α	[76]	1	↓	-	-	-	

(Table 1) contd.....

	Effect	Ref	n	LF	S	I	F	Comment
Pentoxyfylline	suppression of TNF-α gene expression decrease of oxidative stress	[77] [78] [79] [80] [81] [82]	21 26 20 9 20 13	↓ ↓ ↓ ↓ ↓	↓ ↓ ↓ ↓	↓ ↓ ↓ ↓	↓ ↓ ↓ →	oxidized fatty acid level ↓
Losartan	angiotensin II receptor antagonist	[83] [84] [82] [85]	7 75 12 8	→ → ↓ ↓	↓ →	↓ ↓	→ ↓	FFA→ leptin, TNF-α, IL-6, CRP↓ VAT ↓, SAT ↓
Telmisartan	angiotensin II receptor antagonist	[84]	12	→				FFA↓ CT scan: L/S ratio ↑
Resveratrol	antioxidant, insulin sensitizer	[86]	11	↓				HOMA-index, leptin, TNF-α ↓ 1H-MRS: lipid content ↓
Cysteamine bitartrate	antioxidant anti-apoptotic	[87] [88]	11 10	↓ ↓				children, adiponectin ↑, CK-18 fragment↓ adiponectin↑
Betaine	methyldonor antioxidant	[89] [90]	16 10	→ ↓	→ →	→ ↓	→ ↓	S-adenosylmethionine↑
N-acetylcysteine	antioxidant	[91]	15	↓				
Silybin+phosphatidyl-choline+vitamin-E	antioxidant	[92] [93]	53 69	↓	↓	↓	↓	insulin↓, HOMA-index↓ HOMA-index ↓
Probiotics	intestinal bacterial flora	[94] [95] [96]	10 10 22	↓ ↓ ↓				1H-MRS: lipid content ↓ children MDA, 4-HNE ↓

1H-MRS= proton magnetic resonance spectroscopy; 4-HE= 4-hidroxynonenal; F=fibrosis; FFA= free fatty acids; I= inflammation; LF=transaminase activity; MDA=malondialdehyde; N= number of patients; S= steatosis; SAT=subcutaneous adipose tissue; VAT=visceral adipose tissue diameter;

Further controlled clinical studies are needed to establish the real value of the suggested treatment modalities, although these are still in experimental phase. The combination of lifestyle intervention and pharmaceutical therapy targeting main signaling pathways related to lipid metabolism, oxidative stress and inflammation may be combined in the future.

CONFLICT OF INTEREST

The authors confirm that they have no conflict of interest to declare for this publication.

ACKNOWLEDGEMENTS

Declared none.

REFERENCES

[1]   Lomonaco R, Sunny NE, Bril F, Cusi K. Nonalcoholic fatty liver disease: current issues and novel treatment approaches. Drugs 2013; 73(1): 1-14.
        [http://dx.doi.org/10.1007/s40265-012-0004-0] [PMID: 23329465]

[2]   Hagymási K, Lengyel G. [Non-alcoholic steatosis/steatohepatitis 2010]. Orv Hetil 2010; 151(47): 1940-5. [Article in Hungarian].
        [http://dx.doi.org/10.1556/OH.2010.28989] [PMID: 21071305]

[3]   Chalasani N, Younossi Z, Lavine JE, *et al.* The diagnosis and management of non-alcoholic fatty liver disease: Practice guideline by the American Association for the Study of Liver Diseases, American College of Gastroenterology, and the American Gastroenterological Association. Am J Gastroenterol 2012; 107(6): 811-26.
        [http://dx.doi.org/10.1038/ajg.2012.128] [PMID: 22641309]

[4]   Masuoka HC, Chalasani N. Nonalcoholic fatty liver disease: an emerging threat to obese and diabetic individuals. Ann N Y Acad Sci 2013; 1281: 106-22.
        [http://dx.doi.org/10.1111/nyas.12016] [PMID: 23363012]

[5]   Tarantino G, Finelli C. What about non-alcoholic fatty liver disease as a new criterion to define metabolic syndrome? World J Gastroenterol 2013; 19(22): 3375-84.
        [http://dx.doi.org/10.3748/wjg.v19.i22.3375] [PMID: 23801829]

[6]   Vernon G, Baranova A, Younossi ZM. Systematic review: the epidemiology and natural history of non-alcoholic fatty liver disease and non-alcoholic steatohepatitis in adults. Aliment Pharmacol Ther 2011; 34(3): 274-85.
        [http://dx.doi.org/10.1111/j.1365-2036.2011.04724.x] [PMID: 21623852]

[7]   Strauss RS, Barlow SE, Dietz WH. Prevalence of abnormal serum aminotransferase values in overweight and obese adolescents. J Pediatr 2000; 136(6): 727-33.
        [PMID: 10839867]

[8]   Baffy G, Brunt EM, Caldwell SH. Hepatocellular carcinoma in non-alcoholic fatty liver disease: an emerging menace. J Hepatol 2012; 56(6): 1384-91.
        [http://dx.doi.org/10.1016/j.jhep.2011.10.027] [PMID: 22326465]

[9]   Adinolfi LE, Restivo L, Marrone A. The predictive value of steatosis in hepatitis C virus infection. Expert Rev Gastroenterol Hepatol 2013; 7(3): 205-13.
        [http://dx.doi.org/10.1586/egh.13.7] [PMID: 23445230]

[10]   Lakatos M, Hagymási K, Lengyel G. [Fatty liver and hepatitis C virus infection]. Orv Hetil 2011; 152(38): 1513-9.
        [http://dx.doi.org/10.1556/OH.2011.29209] [PMID: 21896442]

[11]   Greenfield V, Cheung O, Sanyal AJ. Recent advances in nonalcoholic fatty liver disease. Curr Opin Gastroenterol 2008; 24(3): 320-7.
        [http://dx.doi.org/10.1097/MOG.0b013e3282fbccf2] [PMID: 18408460]

[12]   Carter-Kent C, Zein NN, Feldstein AE. Cytokines in the pathogenesis of fatty liver and disease progression to steatohepatitis: implications for treatment. Am J Gastroenterol 2008; 103(4): 1036-42.
        [http://dx.doi.org/10.1111/j.1572-0241.2007.01709.x] [PMID: 18177455]

[13]   Cheung O, Sanyal AJ. Recent advances in nonalcoholic fatty liver disease. Curr Opin Gastroenterol 2010; 26(3): 202-8.

[http://dx.doi.org/10.1097/MOG.0b013e328337b0c4] [PMID: 20168226]

[14]   Neuschwander-Tetri BA. Nonalcoholic steatohepatitis and the metabolic syndrome. Am J Med Sci 2005; 330(6): 326-35.
[http://dx.doi.org/10.1097/00000441-200512000-00011] [PMID: 16355018]

[15]   Baffy G. Kupffer cells in non-alcoholic fatty liver disease: the emerging view. J Hepatol 2009; 51(1): 212-23.
[http://dx.doi.org/10.1016/j.jhep.2009.03.008] [PMID: 19447517]

[16]   Carvalho BM, Saad MJ. Influence of Gut Microbiota on Subclinical Inflammation and Insulin Resistance. Mediat Inflamm 2013; 986734.
[http://dx.doi.org/10.1155/2013/986734]

[17]   Yoon HJ, Cha BS. Pathogenesis and therapeutic approaches for non-alcoholic fatty liver disease. World J Hepatol 2014; 6(11): 800-11.
[http://dx.doi.org/10.4254/wjh.v6.i11.800] [PMID: 25429318]

[18]   Dyson JK, Anstee QM, McPherson S. Non-alcoholic fatty liver disease: a practical approach to treatment. Frontline Gastroenterol 2014; 5(4): 277-86.
[http://dx.doi.org/10.1136/flgastro-2013-100404] [PMID: 25285192]

[19]   Tilg H, Moschen AR. Evolving therapies for non-alcoholic steatohepatitis. Expert Opin Drug Discov 2014; 9(6): 687-96.
[http://dx.doi.org/10.1517/17460441.2014.911283] [PMID: 24766298]

[20]   Pearlman M, Loomba R. State of the art: treatment of nonalcoholic steatohepatitis. Curr Opin Gastroenterol 2014; 30(3): 223-37.
[http://dx.doi.org/10.1097/MOG.0000000000000060] [PMID: 24717764]

[21]   Ratziu V, Bellentani S, Cortez-Pinto H, Day C, Marchesini G. A position statement on NAFLD/NASH based on the EASL 2009 special conference. J Hepatol 2010; 53(2): 372-84.
[http://dx.doi.org/10.1016/j.jhep.2010.04.008] [PMID: 20494470]

[22]   Eckard C, Cole R, Lockwood J, *et al.* Prospective histopathologic evaluation of lifestyle modification in nonalcoholic fatty liver disease: a randomized trial. Therap Adv Gastroenterol 2013; 6(4): 249-59.
[http://dx.doi.org/10.1177/1756283X13484078] [PMID: 23814606]

[23]   Méndez-Sánchez N, Arrese M, Zamora-Valdés D, Uribe M. Treating nonalcoholic fatty liver disease. Liver Int 2007; 27(9): 1157-65.
[PMID: 17919226]

[24]   Targher G, Bellis A, Fornengo P, *et al.* Prevention and treatment of nonalcoholic fatty liver disease. Dig Liver Dis 2010; 42(5): 331-40.
[http://dx.doi.org/10.1016/j.dld.2010.02.004] [PMID: 20207207]

[25]   Finelli C, Tarantino G. Is there any consensus as to what diet or lifestyle approach is the right one for NAFLD patients? J Gastrointestin Liver Dis 2012; 21(3): 293-302.
[PMID: 23012671]

[26]   Attar BM, Van Thiel DH. Current concepts and management approaches in nonalcoholic fatty liver disease. Sci Wourld J 2013; 481893.

[27]   Johnston RD, Stephenson MC, Crossland H, *et al.* No difference between high-fructose and high-glucose diets on liver triacylglycerol or biochemistry in healthy overweight men. Gastroenterology 2013; 145(5): 1016-1025.e2.
[http://dx.doi.org/10.1053/j.gastro.2013.07.012] [PMID: 23872500]

[28]   Xu J, Cho H, OMalley S, Park JH, Clarke SD. Dietary polyunsaturated fats regulate rat liver sterol regulatory element binding proteins-1 and -2 in three distinct stages and by different mechanisms. J Nutr 2002; 132(11): 3333-9.

[PMID: 12421847]

[29]   Simopoulos AP. Dietary omega-3 fatty acid deficiency and high fructose intake in the development of metabolic syndrome, brain metabolic abnormalities, and non-alcoholic fatty liver disease. Nutrients 2013; 5(8): 2901-23.
[http://dx.doi.org/10.3390/nu5082901] [PMID: 23896654]

[30]   Scorletti E, Byrne CD. Omega-3 fatty acids, hepatic lipid metabolism, and nonalcoholic fatty liver disease. Annu Rev Nutr 2013; 33: 231-48.
[http://dx.doi.org/10.1146/annurev-nutr-071812-161230] [PMID: 23862644]

[31]   Saab S, Mallam D, Cox I, et al. Impact of coffee on liver diseases: a systematic review. Liver Int 2013.
[http://dx.doi.org/10.1111/liv.12304] [PMID: 24102757]

[32]   Liangpunsakul S, Chalasani N. What should we recommend to our patients with NAFLD regarding alcohol use? Am J Gastroenterol 2012; 107(7): 976-8.
[http://dx.doi.org/10.1038/ajg.2012.20] [PMID: 22764020]

[33]   Baur JA. Biochemical effects of SIRT1 activators. Biochim Biophys Acta 1804; 1804: 1626-34.

[34]   Snow V, Barry P, Fitterman N, Qaseem A, Weiss K. Pharmacologic and surgical management of obesity in primary care: a clinical practice guideline from the American College of Physicians. Ann Intern Med 2005; 142(7): 525-31.
[http://dx.doi.org/10.7326/0003-4819-142-7-200504050-00011] [PMID: 15809464]

[35]   http://sibutramine.com

[36]   Mallat A, Teixeira-Clerc F, Lotersztajn S. Lotersztajn S. Cannabinoid signaling and liver therapeutics. J Hepatol 2013 Apr 6; pii: S0168-8278. (13)00212-2

[37]   Mallat A, Teixeira-Clerc F, Deveaux V, Manin S, Lotersztajn S. The endocannabinoid system as a key mediator during liver diseases: new insights and therapeutic openings. Br J Pharmacol 2011; 163(7): 1432-40.
[http://dx.doi.org/10.1111/j.1476-5381.2011.01397.x] [PMID: 21457226]

[38]   Tam J, Vemuri VK, Liu J, et al. Peripheral CB1 cannabinoid receptor blockade improves cardiometabolic risk in mouse models of obesity. J Clin Invest 2010; 120(8): 2953-66.
[http://dx.doi.org/10.1172/JCI42551] [PMID: 20664173]

[39]   Tam J, Cinar R, Liu J, et al. Peripheral cannabinoid-1 receptor inverse agonism reduces obesity by reversing leptin resistance. Cell Metab 2012; 16(2): 167-79.
[http://dx.doi.org/10.1016/j.cmet.2012.07.002] [PMID: 22841573]

[40]   Holes-Lewis KA, Malcolm R, ONeil PM. Pharmacotherapy of obesity: clinical treatments and considerations. Am J Med Sci 2013; 345(4): 284-8.
[http://dx.doi.org/10.1097/MAJ.0b013e31828abcfd] [PMID: 23531960]

[41]   Athyros VG, Tziomalos K, Karagiannis A, Mikhailidis DP. Cardiovascular benefits of bariatric surgery in morbidly obese patients. Obes Rev 2011; 12(7): 515-24.
[http://dx.doi.org/10.1111/j.1467-789X.2010.00831.x] [PMID: 21348922]

[42]   Mummadi RR, Kasturi KS, Chennareddygari S, Sood GK. Effect of bariatric surgery on nonalcoholic fatty liver disease: systematic review and meta-analysis. Clin Gastroenterol Hepatol 2008; 6(12): 1396-402.
[http://dx.doi.org/10.1016/j.cgh.2008.08.012] [PMID: 18986848]

[43]   Mathurin P, Hollebecque A, Arnalsteen L, et al. Prospective study of the long-term effects of bariatric surgery on liver injury in patients without advanced disease. Gastroenterology 2009; 137(2): 532-40.
[http://dx.doi.org/10.1053/j.gastro.2009.04.052] [PMID: 19409898]

[44]   Defronzo RA, Mehta RJ, Schnure JJ. Pleiotropic effects of thiazolidinediones: implications for the

treatment of patients with type 2 diabetes mellitus. Hosp Pract (1995) 2013; 41(2): 132-47.
[http://dx.doi.org/10.3810/hp.2013.04.1062] [PMID: 23680744]

[45]   Cuthbertson DJ, Irwin A, Gardner CJ, *et al.* Improved glycaemia correlates with liver fat reduction in obese, type 2 diabetes, patients given glucagon-like peptide-1 (GLP-1) receptor agonists. PLoS One 2012; 7(12): e50117.
[http://dx.doi.org/10.1371/journal.pone.0050117] [PMID: 23236362]

[46]   Lee J, Hong SW, Chae SW, *et al.* Exendin-4 improves steatohepatitis by increasing Sirt1 expression in high-fat diet-induced obese C57BL/6J mice. PLoS One 2012; 7(2): e31394.
[http://dx.doi.org/10.1371/journal.pone.0031394] [PMID: 22363635]

[47]   Tushuizen ME, Bunck MC, Pouwels PJ, van Waesberghe JH, Diamant M, Heine RJ. Incretin mimetics as a novel therapeutic option for hepatic steatosis. Liver Int 2006; 26(8): 1015-7.
[http://dx.doi.org/10.1111/j.1478-3231.2006.01315.x] [PMID: 16953843]

[48]   Buse JB, Klonoff DC, Nielsen LL, *et al.* Metabolic effects of two years of exenatide treatment on diabetes, obesity, and hepatic biomarkers in patients with type 2 diabetes: an interim analysis of data from the open-label, uncontrolled extension of three double-blind, placebo-controlled trials. Clin Ther 2007; 29(1): 139-53.
[http://dx.doi.org/10.1016/j.clinthera.2007.01.015] [PMID: 17379054]

[49]   Jendle J, Nauck MA, Matthews DR, *et al.* Weight loss with liraglutide, a once-daily human glucagon-like peptide-1 analogue for type 2 diabetes treatment as monotherapy or added to metformin, is primarily as a result of a reduction in fat tissue. Diabetes Obes Metab 2009; 11(12): 1163-72.
[http://dx.doi.org/10.1111/j.1463-1326.2009.01158.x] [PMID: 19930006]

[50]   Kenny PR, Brady DE, Torres DM, Ragozzino L, Chalasani N, Harrison SA. Exenatide in the treatment of diabetic patients with non-alcoholic steatohepatitis: a case series. Am J Gastroenterol 2010; 105(12): 2707-9.
[http://dx.doi.org/10.1038/ajg.2010.363] [PMID: 21131943]

[51]   Iwasaki T, Yoneda M, Inamori M, *et al.* Sitagliptin as a novel treatment agent for non-alcoholic Fatty liver disease patients with type 2 diabetes mellitus. Hepatogastroenterology 2011; 58(112): 2103-5.
[http://dx.doi.org/10.5754/hge11263] [PMID: 22024083]

[52]   Yilmaz Y, Yonal O, Deyneli O, Celikel CA, Kalayci C, Duman DG. Effects of sitagliptin in diabetic patients with nonalcoholic steatohepatitis. Acta Gastroenterol Belg 2012; 75(2): 240-4.
[PMID: 22870790]

[53]   Ohki T, Isogawa A, Iwamoto M, *et al.* The effectiveness of liraglutide in nonalcoholic fatty liver disease patients with type 2 diabetes mellitus compared to sitagliptin and pioglitazone. Sci W J 2012; 2012: 496453.
[http://dx.doi.org/10.1100/2012/496453]

[54]   Armstrong MJ, Houlihan DD, Rowe IA, *et al.* Safety and efficacy of liraglutide in patients with type 2 diabetes and elevated liver enzymes: individual patient data meta-analysis of the LEAD program. Aliment Pharmacol Ther 2013; 37(2): 234-42.
[http://dx.doi.org/10.1111/apt.12149] [PMID: 23163663]

[55]   Morita Y, Ueno T, Sasaki N, *et al.* Nateglinide is useful for nonalcoholic steatohepatitis (NASH) patients with type 2 diabetes. Hepatogastroenterology 2005; 52(65): 1338-43.
[PMID: 16201069]

[56]   Nseir W, Mahamid M. Statins in nonalcoholic fatty liver disease and steatohepatitis: updated review. Curr Atheroscler Rep 2013; 15(3): 305.
[http://dx.doi.org/10.1007/s11883-012-0305-5] [PMID: 23328905]

[57]   Genuth S, Ismail-Beigi F. Clinical implications of the ACCORD trial. J Clin Endocrinol Metab 2012; 97(1): 41-8.

[http://dx.doi.org/10.1210/jc.2011-1679] [PMID: 22049171]

[58] Basaranoglu M, Acbay O, Sonsuz A. A controlled trial of gemfibrozil in the treatment of patients with nonalcoholic steatohepatitis. J Hepatol 1999; 31(2): 384. [letter].
[http://dx.doi.org/10.1016/S0168-8278(99)80243-8] [PMID: 10453959]

[59] Park H, Shima T, Yamaguchi K, *et al.* Efficacy of long-term ezetimibe therapy in patients with nonalcoholic fatty liver disease. J Gastroenterol 2011; 46(1): 101-7.
[http://dx.doi.org/10.1007/s00535-010-0291-8] [PMID: 20658156]

[60] Enjoji M, Machida K, Kohjima M, *et al.* NPC1L1 inhibitor ezetimibe is a reliable therapeutic agent for non-obese patients with nonalcoholic fatty liver disease. Lipids Health Dis 2010; 9: 29.
[http://dx.doi.org/10.1186/1476-511X-9-29] [PMID: 20222991]

[61] Merat S, Aduli M, Kazemi R, *et al.* Liver histology changes in nonalcoholic steatohepatitis after one year of treatment with probucol. Dig Dis Sci 2008; 53(8): 2246-50.
[http://dx.doi.org/10.1007/s10620-007-0109-6] [PMID: 18049900]

[62] Miller ER III, Pastor-Barriuso R, Dalal D, Riemersma RA, Appel LJ, Guallar E. Meta-analysis: high-dosage vitamin E supplementation may increase all-cause mortality. Ann Intern Med 2005; 142(1): 37-46.
[http://dx.doi.org/10.7326/0003-4819-142-1-200501040-00110] [PMID: 15537682]

[63] Klein EA, Thompson IM Jr, Tangen CM, *et al.* Vitamin E and the risk of prostate cancer. The selenium and vitamin E cancer prevention trial (SELECT). JAMA 2011; 306(14): 1549-56.
[http://dx.doi.org/10.1001/jama.2011.1437] [PMID: 21990298]

[64] Kotb MA. Molecular mechanisms of ursodeoxycholic acid toxicity & side effects: ursodeoxycholic acid freezes regeneration & induces hibernation mode. Int J Mol Sci 2012; 13(7): 8882-914.
[http://dx.doi.org/10.3390/ijms13078882] [PMID: 22942741]

[65] Troisi G, Crisciotti F, Gianturco V, *et al.* The treatment with ursodeoxycholic acid in elderly patients affected by NAFLD and metabolic syndrome: a case-control study. Clin Ter 2013; 164(3): 203-7.
[PMID: 23868620]

[66] Charlton M. Evolving aspects of liver transplantation for nonalcoholic steatohepatitis. Curr Opin Organ Transplant 2013; 18(3): 251-8.
[http://dx.doi.org/10.1097/MOT.0b013e3283615d30] [PMID: 23652610]

[67] Pár G, Horváth G, Pár A. [Non-alcoholic fatty liver disease and steatohepatitis]. Orv Hetil 2013; 154(29): 1124-34. [Non-alcoholic fatty liver disease and steatohepatitis]. [Article in Hungarian].
[http://dx.doi.org/10.1556/OH.2013.29626] [PMID: 23853345]

[68] Afzali A, Berry K, Ioannou GN. Excellent posttransplant survival for patients with nonalcoholic steatohepatitis in the United States. Liver Transpl 2012; 18(1): 29-37.
[http://dx.doi.org/10.1002/lt.22435] [PMID: 21932374]

[69] Kallwitz ER. Metabolic syndrome after liver transplantation: preventable illness or common consequence? World J Gastroenterol 2012; 18(28): 3627-34.
[http://dx.doi.org/10.3748/wjg.v18.i28.3627] [PMID: 22851856]

[70] Malik SM, deVera ME, Fontes P, Shaikh O, Ahmad J. Outcome after liver transplantation for NASH cirrhosis. Am J Transplant 2009; 9(4): 782-93.
[http://dx.doi.org/10.1111/j.1600-6143.2009.02590.x] [PMID: 19344467]

[71] Yalamanchili K, Saadeh S, Klintmalm GB, Jennings LW, Davis GL. Nonalcoholic fatty liver disease after liver transplantation for cryptogenic cirrhosis or nonalcoholic fatty liver disease. Liver Transpl 2010; 16(4): 431-9.
[PMID: 20373454]

[72]   Kelishadi R, Farajian S, Mirlohi M. Probiotics as a novel treatment for non-alcoholic Fatty liver disease; a systematic review on the current evidences. Hepat Mon 2013; 13(4): e7233.
[http://dx.doi.org/10.5812/hepatmon.7233] [PMID: 23885277]

[73]   Lewis JR, Mohanty SR. Nonalcoholic fatty liver disease: a review and update. Dig Dis Sci 2010; 55(3): 560-78.
[http://dx.doi.org/10.1007/s10620-009-1081-0] [PMID: 20101463]

[74]   Musso G, Gambino R, Cassader M. Emerging molecular targets for the treatment of nonalcoholic fatty liver disease. Annu Rev Med 2010; 61: 375-92.
[http://dx.doi.org/10.1146/annurev.med.60.101107.134820] [PMID: 20059344]

[75]   Poulsen MM, Jørgensen JO, Jessen N, Richelsen B, Pedersen SB. Resveratrol in metabolic health: an overview of the current evidence and perspectives. Ann N Y Acad Sci 2013; 1290: 74-82.
[http://dx.doi.org/10.1111/nyas.12141] [PMID: 23855468]

[76]   Schramm C, Schneider A, Marx A, Lohse AW. Adalimumab could suppress the activity of non alcoholic steatohepatitis (NASH). Z Gastroenterol 2008; 46(12): 1369-71.
[http://dx.doi.org/10.1055/s-2008-1027411] [PMID: 19053005]

[77]   Zein CO, Lopez R, Fu X, *et al.* Pentoxifylline decreases oxidized lipid products in nonalcoholic steatohepatitis: new evidence on the potential therapeutic mechanism. Hepatology 2012; 56(4): 1291-9.
[http://dx.doi.org/10.1002/hep.25778] [PMID: 22505276]

[78]   Zein CO, Yerian LM, Gogate P, *et al.* Pentoxifylline improves nonalcoholic steatohepatitis: a randomized placebo-controlled trial. Hepatology 2011; 54(5): 1610-9.
[http://dx.doi.org/10.1002/hep.24544] [PMID: 21748765]

[79]   Van Wagner LB, Koppe SW, Brunt EM, *et al.* Pentoxifylline for the treatment of non-alcoholic steatohepatitis: a randomized controlled trial. Ann Hepatol 2011; 10(3): 277-86.
[PMID: 21677329]

[80]   Satapathy SK, Sakhuja P, Malhotra V, Sharma BC, Sarin SK. Beneficial effects of pentoxifylline on hepatic steatosis, fibrosis and necroinflammation in patients with non-alcoholic steatohepatitis. J Gastroenterol Hepatol 2007; 22(5): 634-8.
[PMID: 17444848]

[81]   Adams LA, Zein CO, Angulo P, Lindor KD. A pilot trial of pentoxifylline in nonalcoholic steatohepatitis. Am J Gastroenterol 2004; 99(12): 2365-8.
[http://dx.doi.org/10.1111/j.1572-0241.2004.40064.x] [PMID: 15571584]

[82]   Georgescu EF, Georgescu M. Therapeutic options in non-alcoholic steatohepatitis (NASH). Are all agents alike? Results of a preliminary study. J Gastrointestin Liver Dis 2007; 16(1): 39-46.
[PMID: 17410287]

[83]   Hirata T, Tomita K, Kawai T, *et al.* Effect of Telmisartan or Losartan for Treatment of Nonalcoholic Fatty Liver Disease: Fatty Liver Protection Trial by Telmisartan or Losartan Study (FANTASY). Int J Endocrinol 2013; 2013: 587140.
[http://dx.doi.org/10.1155/2013/587140] [PMID: 23997767]

[84]   Fogari R, Maffioli P, Mugellini A, Zoppi A, Lazzari P, Derosa G. Effects of losartan and amlodipine alone or combined with simvastatin in hypertensive patients with nonalcoholic hepatic steatosis. Eur J Gastroenterol Hepatol 2012; 24(2): 164-71.
[http://dx.doi.org/10.1097/MEG.0b013e32834ba188] [PMID: 22081005]

[85]   Yokohama S, Yoneda M, Haneda M, *et al.* Therapeutic efficacy of an angiotensin II receptor antagonist in patients with nonalcoholic steatohepatitis. Hepatology 2004; 40(5): 1222-5.
[http://dx.doi.org/10.1002/hep.20420] [PMID: 15382153]

[86] Timmers S, Konings E, Bilet L, *et al.* Calorie restriction-like effects of 30 days of resveratrol supplementation on energy metabolism and metabolic profile in obese humans. Cell Metab 2011; 14(5): 612-22.
[http://dx.doi.org/10.1016/j.cmet.2011.10.002] [PMID: 22055504]

[87] Dohil R, Schmeltzer S, Cabrera BL, *et al.* Enteric-coated cysteamine for the treatment of paediatric non-alcoholic fatty liver disease. Aliment Pharmacol Ther 2011; 33(9): 1036-44.
[http://dx.doi.org/10.1111/j.1365-2036.2011.04626.x] [PMID: 21395631]

[88] Dohil R, Meyer L, Schmeltzer S, Cabrera BL, Lavine JE, Phillips SA. The effect of cysteamine bitartrate on adiponectin multimerization in non-alcoholic fatty liver disease and healthy subjects. J Pediatr 2012; 161(4): 639-45.e1.
[http://dx.doi.org/10.1016/j.jpeds.2012.04.011] [PMID: 22633783]

[89] Abdelmalek MF, Sanderson SO, Angulo P, *et al.* Betaine for nonalcoholic fatty liver disease: results of a randomized placebo-controlled trial. Hepatology 2009; 50(6): 1818-26.
[http://dx.doi.org/10.1002/hep.23239] [PMID: 19824078]

[90] Abdelmalek MF, Angulo P, Jorgensen RA, Sylvestre PB, Lindor KD. Betaine, a promising new agent for patients with nonalcoholic steatohepatitis: results of a pilot study. Am J Gastroenterol 2001; 96(9): 2711-7.
[http://dx.doi.org/10.1111/j.1572-0241.2001.04129.x] [PMID: 11569700]

[91] Pamuk GE, Sonsuz A. N-acetylcysteine in the treatment of non-alcoholic steatohepatitis. J Gastroenterol Hepatol 2003; 18(10): 1220-1.
[http://dx.doi.org/10.1046/j.1440-1746.2003.03156.x] [PMID: 12974918]

[92] Loguercio C, Federico A, Trappoliere M, *et al.* The effect of a silybin-vitamin e-phospholipid complex on nonalcoholic fatty liver disease: a pilot study. Dig Dis Sci 2007; 52(9): 2387-95.
[http://dx.doi.org/10.1007/s10620-006-9703-2] [PMID: 17410454]

[93] Loguercio C, Andreone P, Brisc C, *et al.* Silybin combined with phosphatidylcholine and vitamin E in patients with nonalcoholic fatty liver disease: a randomized controlled trial. Free Radic Biol Med 2012; 52(9): 1658-65.
[http://dx.doi.org/10.1016/j.freeradbiomed.2012.02.008] [PMID: 22343419]

[94] Wong VW, Won GL, Chim AM, *et al.* Treatment of nonalcoholic steatohepatitis with probiotics. A proof-of-concept study. Ann Hepatol 2013; 12(2): 256-62.
[PMID: 23396737]

[95] Vajro P, Mandato C, Licenziati MR, *et al.* Effects of Lactobacillus rhamnosus strain GG in pediatric obesity-related liver disease. J Pediatr Gastroenterol Nutr 2011; 52(6): 740-3.
[http://dx.doi.org/10.1097/MPG.0b013e31821f9b85] [PMID: 21505361]

[96] Loguercio C, Federico A, Tuccillo C, *et al.* Beneficial effects of a probiotic VSL#3 on parameters of liver dysfunction in chronic liver diseases. J Clin Gastroenterol 2005; 39(6): 540-3.
[http://dx.doi.org/10.1097/01.mcg.0000165671.25272.0f] [PMID: 15942443]

CHAPTER 8

Nonalcoholic Fatty Liver Disease and Hepatocellular Carcinoma

György Baffy*

VA Boston Healthcare System and Brigham and Women's Hospital, Harvard Medical School, Boston, Massachusetts, United States of America

Abstract: Hepatocellular carcinoma (HCC) is the most prevalent form of primary liver cancer and the third leading cause of cancer death in the world. HCC has a poor prognosis unless recognized at an early stage, underscoring the importance of prevention. HCC most often develops in cirrhosis associated with chronic viral, toxic, or genetic liver injury. Notably, HCC has a rising incidence in developed societies with an increasing evidence for the role of nonalcoholic fatty liver disease (NAFLD), which has become the most common liver condition mirroring the spread of obesity and type II diabetes. A significant proportion of HCC associated with NAFLD may occur in the absence of advanced fibrosis or cirrhosis, posing a major challenge to cost-efficient risk stratification. Beyond the strong tumorigenic milieu of cirrhosis, molecular mechanisms of hepatocarcinogenesis in NAFLD include adipose tissue expansion with a pro-inflammatory adipokine profile, general and tissue-specific lipotoxicity, and the cell growth promoting effects of elevated insulin levels. Altered gut microbiota and microRNA deregulation may also contribute to HCC development in NAFLD. After reviewing these topics, the chapter provides a brief overview of the clinical characteristics, screening, and novel opportunities in the chemoprevention of NAFLD-related HCC.

Keywords: Adipose expansion, Cancer prevention, Cancer surveillance, Cirrhosis, Cryptogenic cirrhosis, Diabetes, Dysbiosis, Hepatocarcinogenesis, Hepatocellular carcinoma, Hyperinsulinemia, Insulin resistance, Lipotoxicity, microRNA, Nonalcoholic fatty liver disease, Nonalcoholic steatohepatitis, Noncirrhotic cancer, Obesity, Oncogenesis, Proinflammatory adipokines.

INTRODUCTION

Hepatocellular carcinoma (HCC) is the third leading cause of cancer-related

* **Corresponding author György Baffy:** VA Boston Healthcare System, Section of Gastroenterology, 150 S. Huntington Ave., Room 6A-46, Boston, Massachusetts 02130, USA; Email: gbaffy@partners.org

Tatjana Ábel & Gabriella Lengyel (Eds.)
All rights reserved-© 2017 Bentham Science Publishers

mortality, accounting for more than 500,000 deaths per year worldwide [1]. The majority of HCC cases have been associated with cirrhosis due to chronic infection by hepatitis B virus (HBV) or hepatitis C virus (HCV) and toxic injury from excessive alcohol consumption [2]. HCC is one of the few major cancers becoming increasingly common in the US, as the age-adjusted incidence of HCC has grown from 1.5 to 4.9 per 100,000 individuals in the past 30 years [3]. This trend has been linked to the earlier spread of chronic hepatitis C in this country, but nonalcoholic fatty liver disease (NAFLD) is increasingly implicated in the rising HCC prevalence [4 - 6]. It is therefore critical to improve our understanding of the link between NAFLD and HCC.

NAFLD is strongly associated with obesity and related metabolic disorders such as type II diabetes, and it has become the most common liver condition in the US and other developed societies [7 - 10]. NAFLD is a spectrum of liver disorders, ranging from isolated steatosis to nonalcoholic steatohepatitis (NASH) [11, 12]. Within 10 years of duration, NASH is expected to progress into cirrhosis at a rate of 20% and may lead to major complications, such as portal hypertension, liver failure, and hepatocellular carcinoma (HCC) [11, 13]. The risk of HCC is substantial in advanced NAFLD and the yearly incidence of HCC may reach 2% to 4% in NAFLD-cirrhosis [14, 15], which exceeds the 1.5% incidence justifying HCC surveillance by current recommendations [16]. In a recent survey of the US Surveillance, Epidemiology and End Results (SEER) registry across a 6-year period (2004 to 2009), the number of NAFLD-HCC showed a 9% annual increase [17]. Moreover, a recent analysis of the United Network for Organ Sharing (UNOS) database found that the number of liver transplants for HCC related to NASH has quadrupled from 2002 to 2012 and advanced NAFLD is currently the second leading cause of HCC-related liver transplantation [18]. These data indicate an urgent need to find efficient ways of preventing, detecting, and managing the complications of NAFLD progression including the development of HCC. Now that the cure of chronic hepatitis C is within the reach due to the discovery of highly efficient direct acting antiviral agents, it has become imperative to focus on NAFLD as the next frontier in our efforts to halt the rising prevalence of HCC.

RISK FACTORS OF HCC IN NAFLD

Obesity and Diabetes

There is ample evidence that the risk of developing HCC is increased in obesity and associated metabolic disorders. In a large cohort of 900,000 American adults participating the Cancer Prevention Study II, men with a body mass index (BMI) over 35 kg/m² died from liver cancer 4.5-fold more often than their non obese counterparts [19]. Excess body weight increased the risk of liver cancer by 17% for overweight subjects and 89% for the obese in a meta-analysis of 11 cohort studies encompassing over 11,000 individuals [20]. Most of the 26 million Americans currently affected by diabetes have some form of NAFLD and it is estimated that 25% of them have NASH, indicating an increased risk of disease progression to HCC [21, 22]. Indeed, several large US population-based studies indicated that diabetes is an independent risk factor of HCC [23, 24]. In a prospective cohort study based on the computerized national VA database, data on 173,643 Veterans with diabetes and 650,620 Veterans without diabetes with over 10 years of follow-up indicate that diabetes doubled the risk of chronic liver disease and HCC [25]. According to a recent study on almost 7,000 elderly Americans diagnosed with HCC in the SEER-Medicare database, obesity and diabetes have the greatest population-attributable fraction of risk factors for HCC in both males (36.4%) and females (36.7%), which is consistent with the large prevalence of these metabolic conditions in developed societies [26]. Synergistic effects of obesity and diabetes may result in higher rates of HCC [27]. Accordingly, elimination of diabetes and obesity would have a tremendous impact on reducing the incidence of HCC and NAFLD-related mortality.

NAFLD with Advanced Fibrosis

Epidemiological and long-term follow-up studies indicate that HCC may complicate NAFLD-cirrhosis in the absence of viral, toxic, or genetic liver disease [13, 28]. A prospective US study conducted over a period of 10 years found that NAFLD-cirrhosis was complicated by HCC in 10 out of the 149 cases compared to HCV-cirrhosis in which 25 out of the 147 cases developed HCC [29]. In another analysis from the US, cumulative incidence of NAFLD-cirrhosis was 2.6% per year compared to 4.0% per year among patients with HCV cirrhosis [14]. A Japanese study conducted over 5 years found that HCC occurred in 11.3% of patients with NAFLD-cirrhosis compared to 30.5% of patients with HCV-cirrhosis [15]. However, 5-year survival and recurrence rates of HCC for these 2 different etiologies were very similar [30]. These data indicate that the burden of liver cancer in NAFLD-cirrhosis and in cirrhosis due to viral or toxic causes is comparable.

NAFLD without Advanced Fibrosis

Several lines of evidence indicate that HCC may complicate NAFLD in the absence of advanced fibrosis or established cirrhosis. A recent study of a large US health care claims database covering 18 million individuals identified 4,406 cases of HCC in which NAFLD was the most common underlying risk factor (59%) and there was no ICD code for cirrhosis in 54% of these cases [31]. A more recent study analyzed 17,895 HCC cases from the SEER-Medicare database and found that noncirrhotic NAFLD was the only implicated etiology in 5.8% of the cohort, including 186 cases (1%) of HCC complicating pure steatosis [32]. NAFLD was identified as the third most common cause of HCC in a national cohort of 1,500 US Veterans with a significantly lower proportion of cirrhosis (58.3%) among NAFLD-related HCC compared with HCC related to alcohol (72.4%) or chronic HCV infection (85.6%) [33]. In a recent compilation of case reports and case series from across the globe, we found that 28% of all cases of NAFLD-related HCC had an F2 or lesser stage of liver fibrosis [13]. By contrast, an Italian multicenter prospective study found that almost all HCV-related HCC developed in cirrhosis, while advanced fibrosis as assessed by liver biopsy or noninvasive measures was absent in 54% of the 145 NAFLD-related HCC cases [34]. Since the prevalence of noncirrhotic HCC has a large denominator and several long-term follow-up studies indicate that the risk of HCC projected to all stages of NAFLD may not exceed more than 1 out of 3,000 to 4,000 individuals [35, 36]. However, these numbers are predicted to increase with the duration of NAFLD and with the further spread of obesity and diabetes.

Concurrent Chronic Liver Disease

Based on the growing prevalence of obesity and diabetes, NAFLD is likely to develop in the setting of chronic liver disease of other etiologies and further increase the risk of hepatocarcinogenesis. An already higher risk of HCC was doubled among HCV seropositive subjects with a BMI of 30 kg/m^2 or above in a Taiwanese study [37]. In a French cohort of 771 patients diagnosed with cirrhosis linked to HCV and alcohol, clinically manifested diabetes and obesity resulted in an adjusted hazard ratio of 6.0 for HCC [27]. Contribution of metabolic risk factors to the development of HCC is similarly substantial in alcoholic liver disease. A retrospective analysis of almost 20,000 liver explants in the US liver transplantation database identified obesity as an independent predictor of HCC in patients with alcoholic cirrhosis [38]. In a recently published study on a cohort of patients with liver transplantation for alcoholic cirrhosis at a single French medical center, increased risk of HCC was associated with previous history of overweight and diabetes [39]. In a Swedish study of 616 patients diagnosed with HCC, proportion of the metabolic syndrome was significantly higher among patients with alcoholic liver disease (34%) compared to those with alcoholic liver disease co-occurring with HCV infection (10%) or HCV infection alone (13%)

[40]. These observations suggest that obesity and other metabolic disorders may often act as cofactors for hepatocarcinogenesis with other causative factors of chronic liver disease.

MOLECULAR MECHANISMS OF HCC DEVELOPMENT IN NAFLD

Oncogenic Pathways in Cirrhosis

Most cases of NAFLD-related HCC occur in the setting of cirrhosis, which represents a unique and strong tumorigenic microenvironment [41]. It is well established that cirrhosis is by far the most important risk factor of HCC, with parallel hepatocellular destruction and proliferation in which virtually every major oncogenic pathway such as genomic alterations, epigenetic activation and silencing, and aberrant cascades of intracellular signal transduction [42 - 45]. Development of HCC in cirrhosis usually takes many years with stepwise changes along a dysplasia-carcinoma sequence similarly implicated in several other cancers [46 - 48]. Monitoring of this molecular evolution in the cirrhotic liver is fundamentally important for prognostication and timely intervention [49]. While the unusual molecular heterogeneity of HCC may offer pharmacological targets for different subsets of patients [50, 51], they also account for the level of robustness, high chemoresistance, and poor overall prognosis [52].

Genetic Variability and Predisposition to NAFLD-HCC

While environmental factors play a fundamental role in the pathogenesis of obesity-related disorders including the progression of NAFLD into HCC, genetic predisposition to these conditions has been the subject of intense research. Obesity is a complex condition in which the interplay of many genes and their variants may modulate the phenotype [53, 54]. In a recent report, the Genetic Investigation of Anthropometric Traits (GIANT) consortium described a total of 97 gene regions, 56 of which are entirely novel, in association with obesity [55]. Another genome-wide association study from the same group has identified 49 loci of single nucleotide polymorphism (SNP) linked to body fat distribution, which is an established predictor of adverse metabolic outcomes [56].

SNPs in genes influencing lipid metabolism, insulin signaling, and oxidative stress are likely to modulate individual susceptibility to transition from steatosis to NASH and from NASH to HCC [57]. One of the most investigated SNPs linked to the progression of NAFLD is the I148M sequence variant of the PNPLA3 gene, encoding for adiponutrin involved in hepatocellular lipid processing that has been linked to liver disease of other etiologies, in addition to an increased risk of HCC

[58]. More recent genomic and metabolomic profiling of livers of healthy controls and patients with various stages of NAFLD found that most differences occur during the progression of steatosis to NASH, including the upregulation of genes involved in extracellular matrix formation and angiogenesis [59]. While many of these genes are also upregulated in HCC, early changes in their expression during NASH indicate that they do not represent unique events in the transition from NASH to HCC [59, 60]. Intriguingly, these studies also concluded that loss of steatosis in NASH (*i.e.*, progression to cryptogenic cirrhosis) does not play an important role in development of HCC [59]. Another recent work mapped changes between steatosis and NASH by global microarray gene analysis and found the upregulation of two genes considered as pre-malignant biomarkers (keratene multigene family member KRT23 and the aldose reductase AKR1B10), further supporting the importance of early transition from steatosis to NASH in hepatocarcinogenesis [61].

Recent work indicates that a loss-of-function variant of the transmembrane 6 superfamily member 2 (TM6SF2) gene is associated with an increased risk of developing hepatic lipid deposition and subsequent clinical outcomes [62]. The rs58542926 variant of TM6SF2 contains a glutamate-to-lysine substitution (E167K), which appears to provide protection from atherosclerosis due to lower levels of circulating lipids while it paradoxically results in the accumulation of hepatocellular lipid droplets leading to steatosis [62, 63]. TM6SF2 has been implicated in the biology of very low-density lipoproteins (VLDLs) and experimental findings suggest that it is required to mobilize and package neutral lipids into VLDL assembly but not for VLDL secretion [64]. While there is no evidence for the direct involvement of TM6SF2 polymorphism in NAFLD-associated hepatocarcinogenesis, the rs58542926 variant has recently been linked to an increased risk for HCC in patients with alcoholic cirrhosis [65]. Additional research is needed to gain better understanding of the genetic link between obesity, NAFLD, and HCC.

Adipose Expansion and Adipokine Imbalance

Obesity reflects the sustained imbalance between energy intake and expenditure, which most often corresponds to a mismatch of chronic nutrient excess and diminished physical exercise [53]. Storage of the surplus energy in peripheral adipose tissue promotes tissue remodeling, which involves adipocyte growth and differentiation, recruitment of macrophages and endothelial precursor cells, stimulation of angiogenesis, and a pro-inflammatory adipokine secretion profile [66, 67].

The low-grade, systemic inflammation associated with adipose tissue remodeling can contribute to hepatocarcinogenesis in many ways [68 - 70]. The long list of adipokines, cytokines, and other bioactive substances produced by the numerous cellular components of expanding adipose tissue includes leptin, resistin, visfatin, interleukin (IL)-1β, IL-6, tumor necrosis factor (TNF)-α, plasminogen activator inhibitor-1, macrophage migration inhibitory factor, matrix metalloproteinases (*e.g.*, MMP2 and MMP9), vascular endothelial growth factor, hypoxia-inducible factor-α, and various CXC and CC chemokines [71, 72]. The cellular effects of leptin mostly occur through activation of phosphoinositide 3-kinase (PI3K)/Akt, extracellular signal-regulated kinases (ERKs), and the Janus kinase (JAK)/signal transducer and activator of transcription (STAT) [73]. The permissive effect of adipose-derived TNF-α and IL-6 in diethyl nitrosamine (DEN)-induced liver tumor formation has been well documented [74]. Certain adipose depots may also secrete large amounts of sex-steroid hormones (estrogens, progesterone, and androgens) [19]. Relative lack of adiponectin, a strong activator of 5'-adenosine monophosphate activated protein kinase (AMPK), results in diminished suppression of tumor growth and increased cell apoptosis due to failed inhibition of the mammalian target of rapamycin (mTOR) pathway and c-Jun N-terminal kinase (JNK)/caspase 3 pathways [75].

Lipotoxicity

The liver is the primary site exposed to the pathological effects of excess lipid storage in obesity [76]. Hepatic fat accumulation in NAFLD originates from peripheral fat depots due to insufficient storage capacity or increased release by uncontrolled lipolysis, from the portal vein due to increased dietary intake, and from deregulation of hepatocellular lipid metabolism including increased *de novo* lipogenesis, impaired elimination through fatty acid oxidation, and diminished export of very low-density lipoproteins [77 - 79]. *De novo* lipogenesis is a particularly important component of obesity-associated steatosis. High insulin levels stimulate, and low adiponectin levels fail to block, the lipogenic effects of steroid response element binding protein SREBP-1c and carbohydrate-responsive element-binding protein ChREBP-β [80 - 84]. Moreover, stimulation of lipogenic transactivators such as liver X receptor α (LXRα), peroxisome proliferator-activated receptor γ (PPARγ), and adipocyte lipid-binding protein (AP2) may create cycles of self-perpetuation [85].

Liver steatosis may lead to lipotoxicity, which is defined as chronic cellular and tissue damage related to ectopic lipid accumulation [76, 86, 87]. Lipotoxicity has been associated with mitochondrial dysfunction, oxidative injury, endoplasmic reticulum stress, hepatocellular injury, liver inflammatory response, and suppressed insulin signaling [76, 86, 88, 89]. These mechanisms provide multiple links between the lipotoxicity and hepatocarcinogenesis. Lipotoxicity is associated with lipid peroxidation that may cause oxidative damage in genomic DNA [90]. Lipid constituents may activate various oncogenic pathways by altering the mechanisms of cell signaling and gene transcription [91, 92]. Lipotoxicity may promote the innate immune response through pathways of damage-associated molecular patterns (DAMPs) with the activation of Kupffer cells [93]. Various experimental models provided evidence that NF-κB and other pathways of cell proliferation are stimulated by resident and recruited macrophages in hepatocytes surviving their injury, playing therefore a key role in hepatocarcinogenesis [94, 95]. The primary importance of ectopic fat accumulation and lipotoxicity in hepatocarcinogenesis has been illustrated in mice deficient for the histone reader Trim24, a member of the tripartite motif (TRIM) protein family with a role in cellular differentiation, development, and apoptosis [96]. Trim24 deficiency leads to a striking loss of peripheral fat depots, elevated levels of circulating triglycerides, and steatohepatitis culminating in the spontaneous development of HCC in the absence of obesity [96]. Additional work on this model may provide useful information about the progression of NAFLD to HCC in non-obese individuals.

Insulin Resistance

One of the fundamental mechanisms underlying the pathogenesis of obesity-associated disorders is systemic and hepatic insulin resistance [97]. Lipotoxicity may cause multiple defects in the robust cellular signaling network required for the complex effects of insulin [76, 86, 97]. These changes occur in all tissues that normally respond to insulin and promote compensatory hyperinsulinemia [76, 86, 97]. Sustained high levels of insulin promote the secretion of insulin-like growth factor (IGF)-binding protein and increase the bioavailability of IGF1 and IGF2, further stimulating cellular signaling through PI3K/Akt, mitogen-activated protein kinase (MAPK), and vascular endothelial growth factor (VEGF) [98]. There is experimental evidence that elevated levels of circulating insulin may induce the development of HCC by activating these oncogenic pathways, involving mechanisms that possibly account for the contribution of diabetes to hepatocarcinogenesis independent of obesity [99, 100]. The recent model of chemical hepatocarcinogenesis in NAFLD promoted by choline-deficient L-amino-acid-deficient diet (CDAA) associated with insulin resistance in the absence of cirrhosis may help understand the role of hyperinsulinemia in the development of noncirrhotic HCC [101].

Altered Gut Microbiota

A large number of microorganisms live in mutual coexistence with humans and contribute to various physiological functions. This diverse community, now termed human microbiota, may change dynamically in response to the external environment and their unfavorable alterations (dysbiosis) are linked to various lifestyle and health conditions such as high-fat diet and obesity [102, 103]. Characteristic changes in the composition of gut microbiota in response to obesity have been associated with the progression of NAFLD [104]. There is evidence that increased translocation of intestinal bacteria may contribute to the liver inflammatory response and promote the development of HCC [105]. Recognition of the Gram-negative bacterial cell wall component lipopolysaccharide (LPS) by Toll-like receptor 4 (TLR4) may activate various inflammatory and oncogenic pathways involving TNF-α and IL-6 secretion [94, 106]. Recent work suggests that stellate cells are also involved in this process through TLR4-dependent secretion of growth factors such as epiregulin [107]. The role of gut-derived LPS in hepatocarcinogenesis has been further supported by observations that elimination of the gut microbiota by antibiotics or inhibition of the TLR4 signaling pathway results in diminished tumor growth in the chronically injured liver [107, 108].

A recent study provided intriguing additional information about the link between high-fat diet, gut microbiota, and the development of HCC [108]. In a murine model of chemical hepatocarcinogenesis, high-fat diet increased the rate of liver tumors induced by 7,12-dimethylbenz(a)anthracene (DMBA) in association with dominance of *Clostridium* in the gut microbiota and increased circulating levels of deoxycholic acid (DCA), a secondary bile acid produced by *Clostridium* [108]. These findings identify the gut microbiota as a key contributor to the risk of HCC in NAFLD.

MicroRNAs and Hepatocarcinogenesis

MicroRNAs (miRNAs) are short noncoding RNAs involved in the post-transcriptional regulation of gene expression [109]. There is increasing evidence that miRNAs control many aspects of lipid metabolism, cell proliferation, and apoptosis [110, 111]. Based on experimental models and human observations, various miRNA species have been linked to specific aspects of hepatocarcinogenesis such as metastasis, disease recurrence, and poor prognosis [112 - 114]. miR-122 is the predominant miRNA in adult human liver, regulating hepatic cholesterol metabolism and ER-associated lipid droplet production [115]. Expression of miR-122 is decreased in liver tissue affected by steatosis and HCC formation, suggesting a potential tumor suppressor role of this molecule [116]. miR-34a becomes particularly abundant in NAFLD and it has been shown to regulate hepatic lipid metabolism through a number of targets, including PPARs, PPARγ-coactivator (PGC)-1α, LXR, farnesoid X receptor (FXR), SIRT1, and SREBP-1c [117 - 119]. Remarkably, miR-34a is a direct transcriptional target of the tumor suppressor p53, one of the most frequently mutated genes in HCC [120, 121]. On the other hand, p53 function is impaired through the blockade of its positive regulator HPB1, which is a target of miR-21, another miRNA found to be upregulated in human HCC [122].

Additional miRNA species involved in lipid metabolism include miR-370 and the miR-122 activator miR-33a/b, while miR-99b and miR-197 have been linked to visceral adipose tissue in NAFLD patients and found to be significantly associated with pericellular fibrosis [123 - 125]. Several authors suggest that different miRNA signatures may help in distinguishing the contribution of obesity-associated factors from other etiologies in the development of HCC [117, 118, 126]. Better understanding of the overlapping miRNA regulation in lipid metabolism and hepatocarcinogenesis may support new ways of prognostication and therapy for HCC [127].

DIAGNOSIS OF NAFLD-HCC

Clinical Presentation

NAFLD-related HCC diagnosed with or without cirrhosis may have different imaging and pathological features including size, differentiation, and encapsulation [128, 129]. Most cases of NAFLD-related HCC occur as a solitary large mass and remain well differentiated despite the larger size [130, 131]. Consistent with the observations that an increasing proportion of NAFLD-related HCC occurs in noncirrhotic livers, these morphological features are characteristically seen in malignant liver lesions that develop amidst mild or no fibrosis [132 - 134]. In a French study of 31 patients with HCC linked to the metabolic syndrome, stage F0-F2 fibrosis was associated with an average tumor diameter of 10.1 cm, whereas the average size of cirrhosis-associated tumors was 6.6 cm [128]. Similarly, a recent study on 54 patients with NAFLD-related HCC from Australia found that HCC nodules in noncirrhotic patients had significantly larger diameter at the time of diagnosis compared to those associated with cirrhosis (4.7 cm *vs.* 3.2 cm) [135]. While noncirrhotic HCC cases have a generally better prognosis and may be amenable to more aggressive therapeutic opportunities in the absence of significant background liver disease, larger tumor size at least partially accounts for the fact that a greater proportion of noncirrhotic patients in the aforementioned Australian study failed the Milan criteria for transplantation (87.5% *vs.* 28.2%) [135].

Biomarkers of HCC Development in NAFLD

The most studied serum biomarkers of HCC include alpha-fetoprotein (AFP) and des-carboxyprothrombin (DCP). However, these biomarkers have less than desirable sensitivity and do not predict the development of HCC in NAFLD [136 - 138]. The utility of AFP in HCC surveillance remains controversial [139 - 141]. There is an intense search for novel genetic, epigenetic, proteomic, and metabolic biomarkers that may offer early diagnosis of HCC, provide useful information according to specific etiologies, predict an increased risk of hepatocarcinogenesis in the noncirrhotic liver, associate with the progression of dysplastic liver lesions, distinguish multicentric HCC from intrahepatic metastases, and indicate the risk of tumor recurrence [49, 59, 142 - 144]. Regrettably, there are currently no such biomarkers available. Circulating miRNAs currently represent a promising group of molecules as noninvasive diagnostic markers to follow the progression of NAFLD and the development of HCC [127]. It is our hope that the relentless evolution of systems biology, network-based approaches such as gene-enrichment analysis, computational gene prioritization, and new function assignment through guilt-by-association will soon offer novel tools for the more efficient prevention and diagnosis of NAFLD-related HCC [145].

RISK REDUCTION STRATEGIES FOR HCC COMPLICATING NAFLD

Screening and Surveillance

Timely recognition of HCC that complicates the course of NAFLD is a challenging task for several reasons. As discussed before, HCC may develop before cirrhosis and there are no established screening guidelines for noncirrhotic HCC due to the prohibitive costs of finding a rare event in an exceedingly large population [13, 146]. On the other hand, NAFLD is recognized as a major cause of cryptogenic cirrhosis, a condition in which most histological features of NAFLD may have disappeared and the medical history supporting a metabolic etiology could be long forgotten [147, 148]. This is a major concern since cryptogenic cirrhosis in developed societies is associated with up to 40% of HCC cases diagnosed without other obvious risk factors [6]. The problem has been well illustrated by a US single-center study in which HCC associated with cryptogenic cirrhosis was significantly more often discovered by clinical symptoms than by surveillance [149]. According to a more recent retrospective study based on a national cohort of VA hospitals, 56.7% of patients with NAFLD-related HCC did not receive surveillance in the 3 years prior to their HCC diagnosis, compared to patients with alcohol-related (40.2%) or HCV-related HCC (13.3%) and this difference persisted in the proportion of patients receiving HCC-specific treatment [33]. A recent report from the Karolinska University Hospital in Sweden indicates that the problem of delayed HCC diagnosis in NAFLD knows no geographical boundaries [40]. This retrospective analysis of 616 patients diagnosed with HCC found that no surveillance was performed in 36% of cases associated with NAFLD compared to only 7.5-14% in patients with hepatitis C with or without concurrent alcoholic liver disease. Not surprisingly, survival was significantly better in patients who underwent surveillance compared with those in whom surveillance was missed in the absence of known liver disease, most of them diagnosed with metabolic derangements such as obesity, diabetes, and hypertension [40]. This lesson was echoed by the recent SEER survey in which patients with NAFLD-HCC were older, had shorter survival time, and were more likely to die from their primary liver cancer [17]. These findings indicate an urgent need to develop practical and cost-efficient strategies for identifying individuals with obesity and associated metabolic disorders such as diabetes at increased risk of HCC development and in need of cancer surveillance.

Lifestyle Measures

A number of lifestyle factors, such as increased dietary intake of n-6 polyunsaturated fatty acids or reduced level of fitness, have been associated with the severity of NAFLD [150, 151]. By extension, correction of these measures is likely to reduce the risk of HCC in these individuals, although the extent to which the chance of developing HCC in NAFLD may diminish remains to be seen. Several large-scale epidemiological studies on the effects of bariatric surgery provided evidence that cancer prevention benefits can be expected from 10% to 30% weight loss sustained over 10 years, although it remains unclear if this benefit includes a lower risk of NAFLD-related HCC [152, 153]. Notwithstanding, recent work on hepatocyte-specific PTEN-deficient mice indicates that the number of malignant liver lesions following the administration of high-fat diet for 32 weeks was significantly smaller in a group that had daily 60 minutes of exercise on a motorized treadmill compared to 'sedentary' controls (71% *vs.* 100%) [154]. There is limited information available about the potential impact of dietary factors on the risk of HCC. A recent meta-analysis of 19 eligible studies published on the subject since 1956 found that the risk of HCC may decrease by 8% for every 100 grams of vegetable consumed on a daily basis [155]. Recall bias with the use of questionnaires is a significant concern and additional well-designed and long-term studies will be necessary to confirm these findings.

Insulin-sensitizing Agents

Multiple studies suggest that the risk of HCC is reduced by the use of insulin-sensitizing agents such as metformin and thiazolidinediones, whereas the insulin-secretagogue sulfonylureas and insulin may have an opposing effect [27, 156, 157]. Although diabetes duration and severity may have a confounding effect on these observations, the epidemiological and experimental evidence for the impact of metformin on HCC development seems particularly noteworthy [158]. A retrospective case control study from Italy analyzed 610 cases of diabetes-associated HCC and described an odds ratio of 0.16 for developing HCC among patients treated with metformin compared to those treated with sulfonylureas or insulin [156]. In another study, prospective monitoring of 100 French patients with diabetes and chronic hepatitis C found that 5-year incidence of HCC was 9.5% in patients who received metformin compared to an incidence of 31.2% among those who did not [27]. In a case control study conducted at a large US cancer center, the adjusted odds ratio for HCC was 0.3 among diabetics taking metformin of thiazolidinediones, while it was over 7.0 for those taking insulin secretagogues or relying on dietary control only [159].

Several molecular mechanisms have been proposed to account for the activity of metformin as a cancer preventive agent [158, 160]. The primary action of metformin is linked to activation of AMPK, which not only regulates cellular energy metabolism but also has molecular targets such as the mTOR pathway and the retinoblastoma protein [161]. Metformin inhibits complex I of the mitochondrial respiratory chain and provides an additional uncoupling effect, which may relieve the oxidative stress associated with the high-glucose environment associated with diabetes [162]. Paradoxically, several studies reported that metformin has little or no impact on the progression of NAFLD [163, 164]. The chemopreventive effects of metformin are therefore not necessarily linked to the prevention of steatosis and steatohepatitis, but it may possibly act through the efficient mitigation of prolonged hyperinsulinemia. Future trials that address the bias of diabetes severity in the different use of metformin and may involve safer and more efficient derivatives of metformin will hopefully provide elucidation in this important field.

Emerging Opportunities for Chemoprevention

A significant body of evidence indicates that the 3-hydroxy-3-methylglutaryl coenzyme A reductase inhibitor statins widely utilized to treat dyslipidemia and improve cardiovascular morbidity may have a role in diminishing the risk of HCC. A recent systematic review and meta-analysis encompassing almost 4,300 cases of HCC found that statin users were less likely to develop HCC than non-users and this benefit was particularly apparent in the Asian population (adjusted odds ratio, 0.52) [165]. Subsequent data from a single US health care system indicate that statins may reduce the risk of HCC without a clear dose-response relationship [166]. However, a most recent analysis of the SEER database found that statin use was not associated with improved survival among the 1,036 cases of early-stage HCC diagnosed between 2007 and 2009 [167]. Further research may confirm or refute these data and clarify the mechanism by which lipid-lowering therapy may prevent the onset or slow the progression of HCC in NAFLD.

Farnesoid X receptor (FXR) is a nuclear hormone receptor primarily implicated in bile acid sensing and highly expressed in the liver [168, 169]. As a regulator of gene expression, FXR exerts a number of molecular effects in lipid and glucose metabolism, liver regeneration, inflammation, and cancer [168, 170, 171]. The importance of FXR in cancer prevention has been suggested in FXR-deficient mice that develop HCC and other malignancies [172, 173]. In addition, FXR is downregulated in human HCC, further supporting its protective role in hepatocarcinogenesis [173]. FXR has been shown to inhibit gankyrin, a proteasome factor that promotes the degradation of several tumor suppressor proteins [174]. These observations suggest that pharmacological modulation of FXR may prove to be a promising approach in the prevention and treatment of HCC.

Interestingly, obeticholic acid (6-ethylchenodeoxycholic acid), a synthetic and potent FXR agonist, has recently been shown to improve the histological features of NASH in a 72-week randomized placebo-controlled trial (FLINT) of 283 patients from 8 centers of the US NASH Clinical Research Network [175]. However, the outcomes of FLINT have been received with a somewhat tempered enthusiasm due to the modest histological effects accompanied by pruritus, unwanted changes in the serum lipid profile, and transient increase in hepatic insulin resistance, indicating that FXR has a complex biology and additional studies are needed to confirm the benefits of obeticholic acid in NAFLD [175].

PERSPECTIVES

HCC is one of the most common cancers in the world with one of the poorest prognoses among major malignancies. In addition, HCC is one of the few cancers with an increasing incidence in the US, which is quite concerning at a time when chronic hepatitis C as the primary cause of HCC in this country is going to be (hopefully) soon eliminated due to the rapidly emerging and powerful direct acting antiviral (DAA) therapies. We are now left with NAFLD as an exceedingly common and heterogeneous liver condition linked to the development of HCC. In a minority of patients, NAFLD is advanced to cirrhosis and the yearly incidence of HCC surpasses the threshold of cost-effectiveness for cancer surveillance. In the vast majority, however, NAFLD is mostly benign and the progression to HCC remains rare and seemingly random, obviously not amenable for screening without prior risk stratification. The really big problem is that this scenario involves a quarter of the American populace. It is therefore critical to understand the key molecular drivers of hepatocarcinogenesis associated with NAFLD, obesity, and diabetes to develop financially viable and practical strategies for identifying the targets of effective and large-scale prevention, recognition, and treatment of NAFLD-related HCC.

CONFLICT OF INTEREST

The author confirms that author has no conflict of interest to declare for this publication.

ACKNOWLEDGEMENTS

Declared none.

REFERENCES

[1]   Jemal A, Bray F, Center MM, Ferlay J, Ward E, Forman D. Global cancer statistics. CA Cancer J Clin 2011; 61(2): 69-90.
[http://dx.doi.org/10.3322/caac.20107] [PMID: 21296855]

[2]   El-Serag HB. Hepatocellular carcinoma. N Engl J Med 2011; 365(12): 1118-27.
[http://dx.doi.org/10.1056/NEJMra1001683] [PMID: 21992124]

[3]   Altekruse SF, McGlynn KA, Reichman ME. Hepatocellular carcinoma incidence, mortality, and survival trends in the United States from 1975 to 2005. J Clin Oncol 2009; 27(9): 1485-91.
[http://dx.doi.org/10.1200/JCO.2008.20.7753] [PMID: 19224838]

[4]   Bosch FX, Ribes J, Cléries R, Díaz M. Epidemiology of hepatocellular carcinoma. Clin Liver Dis 2005; 9(2): 191-211, v. [v.].
[http://dx.doi.org/10.1016/j.cld.2004.12.009] [PMID: 15831268]

[5]   Charlton M. Cirrhosis and liver failure in nonalcoholic fatty liver disease: Molehill or mountain? Hepatology 2008; 47(5): 1431-3.
[http://dx.doi.org/10.1002/hep.22246] [PMID: 18393323]

[6]   El-Serag HB, Rudolph KL. Hepatocellular carcinoma: epidemiology and molecular carcinogenesis. Gastroenterology 2007; 132(7): 2557-76.
[http://dx.doi.org/10.1053/j.gastro.2007.04.061] [PMID: 17570226]

[7] Bellentani S, Saccoccio G, Masutti F, *et al.* Prevalence of and risk factors for hepatic steatosis in Northern Italy. Ann Intern Med 2000; 132(2): 112-7.
[http://dx.doi.org/10.7326/0003-4819-132-2-200001180-00004] [PMID: 10644271]

[8] Browning JD, Szczepaniak LS, Dobbins R, *et al.* Prevalence of hepatic steatosis in an urban population in the United States: impact of ethnicity. Hepatology 2004; 40(6): 1387-95.
[http://dx.doi.org/10.1002/hep.20466] [PMID: 15565570]

[9] Chitturi S, Farrell GC, Hashimoto E, Saibara T, Lau GK, Sollano JD. Non-alcoholic fatty liver disease in the Asia-Pacific region: definitions and overview of proposed guidelines. J Gastroenterol Hepatol 2007; 22(6): 778-87.
[http://dx.doi.org/10.1111/j.1440-1746.2007.05001.x] [PMID: 17565630]

[10] Liu CJ. Prevalence and risk factors for non-alcoholic fatty liver disease in Asian people who are not obese. J Gastroenterol Hepatol 2012; 27(10): 1555-60.
[http://dx.doi.org/10.1111/j.1440-1746.2012.07222.x] [PMID: 22741595]

[11] Angulo P. Nonalcoholic fatty liver disease. N Engl J Med 2002; 346(16): 1221-31.
[http://dx.doi.org/10.1056/NEJMra011775] [PMID: 11961152]

[12] Torres DM, Williams CD, Harrison SA. Features, diagnosis, and treatment of nonalcoholic fatty liver disease. Clin Gastroenterol Hepatol 2012; 10(8): 837-58.
[http://dx.doi.org/10.1016/j.cgh.2012.03.011] [PMID: 22446927]

[13] Baffy G, Brunt EM, Caldwell SH. Hepatocellular carcinoma in non-alcoholic fatty liver disease: an emerging menace. J Hepatol 2012; 56(6): 1384-91.
[http://dx.doi.org/10.1016/j.jhep.2011.10.027] [PMID: 22326465]

[14] Ascha MS, Hanouneh IA, Lopez R, Tamimi TA, Feldstein AF, Zein NN. The incidence and risk factors of hepatocellular carcinoma in patients with nonalcoholic steatohepatitis. Hepatology 2010; 51(6): 1972-8.
[http://dx.doi.org/10.1002/hep.23527] [PMID: 20209604]

[15] Yatsuji S, Hashimoto E, Tobari M, Taniai M, Tokushige K, Shiratori K. Clinical features and outcomes of cirrhosis due to non-alcoholic steatohepatitis compared with cirrhosis caused by chronic hepatitis C. J Gastroenterol Hepatol 2009; 24(2): 248-54.
[http://dx.doi.org/10.1111/j.1440-1746.2008.05640.x] [PMID: 19032450]

[16] Sherman M. Hepatocellular carcinoma: screening and staging. Clin Liver Dis 2011; 15(2): 323-334, vii-x. [vii-x.].
[http://dx.doi.org/10.1016/j.cld.2011.03.003] [PMID: 21689616]

[17] Younossi ZM, Otgonsuren M, Henry L, *et al.* Association of nonalcoholic fatty liver disease (NAFLD) with hepatocellular carcinoma (HCC) in the United States from 2004 to 2009. Hepatology 2015; 62(6): 1723-30.
[http://dx.doi.org/10.1002/hep.28123] [PMID: 26274335]

[18] Wong RJ, Cheung R, Ahmed A. Nonalcoholic steatohepatitis is the most rapidly growing indication for liver transplantation in patients with hepatocellular carcinoma in the U.S. Hepatology. Hepatology 2014; 59: 2188-95.

[19] Calle EE, Rodriguez C, Walker-Thurmond K, Thun MJ. Overweight, obesity, and mortality from cancer in a prospectively studied cohort of U.S. adults. N Engl J Med 2003; 348(17): 1625-38.
[http://dx.doi.org/10.1056/NEJMoa021423] [PMID: 12711737]

[20] Larsson SC, Wolk A. Overweight, obesity and risk of liver cancer: a meta-analysis of cohort studies. Br J Cancer 2007; 97(7): 1005-8.
[PMID: 17700568]

[21] Byrne CD, Olufadi R, Bruce KD, Cagampang FR, Ahmed MH. Metabolic disturbances in non-alcoholic fatty liver disease. Clin Sci 2009; 116(7): 539-64.
[http://dx.doi.org/10.1042/CS20080253] [PMID: 19243311]

[22] Williams CD, Stengel J, Asike MI, *et al.* Prevalence of nonalcoholic fatty liver disease and nonalcoholic steatohepatitis among a largely middle-aged population utilizing ultrasound and liver biopsy: a prospective study. Gastroenterology 2011; 140(1): 124-31.
[http://dx.doi.org/10.1053/j.gastro.2010.09.038] [PMID: 20858492]

[23] Davila JA, Morgan RO, Shaib Y, McGlynn KA, El-Serag HB. Diabetes increases the risk of hepatocellular carcinoma in the United States: a population based case control study. Gut 2005; 54(4): 533-9.
[http://dx.doi.org/10.1136/gut.2004.052167] [PMID: 15753540]

[24] El-Serag HB, Hampel H, Javadi F. The association between diabetes and hepatocellular carcinoma: a systematic review of epidemiologic evidence. Clin Gastroenterol Hepatol 2006; 4(3): 369-80.
[http://dx.doi.org/10.1016/j.cgh.2005.12.007] [PMID: 16527702]

[25] El-Serag HB, Tran T, Everhart JE. Diabetes increases the risk of chronic liver disease and hepatocellular carcinoma. Gastroenterology 2004; 126(2): 460-8.
[http://dx.doi.org/10.1053/j.gastro.2003.10.065] [PMID: 14762783]

[26] Welzel TM, Graubard BI, Quraishi S, *et al.* Population-attributable fractions of risk factors for hepatocellular carcinoma in the United States. Am J Gastroenterol 2013; 108(8): 1314-21.
[http://dx.doi.org/10.1038/ajg.2013.160] [PMID: 23752878]

[27] NKontchou G, Paries J, Htar MT, *et al.* Risk factors for hepatocellular carcinoma in patients with alcoholic or viral C cirrhosis. Clin Gastroenterol Hepatol 2006; 4(8): 1062-8.
[http://dx.doi.org/10.1016/j.cgh.2006.05.013] [PMID: 16844421]

[28] Hashimoto E, Tokushige K. Hepatocellular carcinoma in non-alcoholic steatohepatitis: Growing evidence of an epidemic? Hepatol Res 2012; 42(1): 1-14.
[http://dx.doi.org/10.1111/j.1872-034X.2011.00872.x] [PMID: 21917086]

[29] Sanyal AJ, Banas C, Sargeant C, *et al.* Similarities and differences in outcomes of cirrhosis due to nonalcoholic steatohepatitis and hepatitis C. Hepatology 2006; 43(4): 682-9.
[http://dx.doi.org/10.1002/hep.21103] [PMID: 16502396]

[30] Tokushige K, Hashimoto E, Kodama K. Hepatocarcinogenesis in non-alcoholic fatty liver disease in Japan. J Gastroenterol Hepatol 2013; 28 (Suppl. 4): 88-92.
[http://dx.doi.org/10.1111/jgh.12239] [PMID: 24251711]

[31] Sanyal A, Poklepovic A, Moyneur E, Barghout V. Population-based risk factors and resource utilization for HCC: US perspective. Curr Med Res Opin 2010; 26(9): 2183-91.
[http://dx.doi.org/10.1185/03007995.2010.506375] [PMID: 20666689]

[32] Rahman RN, Ibdah JA. Nonalcoholic fatty liver disease without cirrhosis is an emergent and independent risk factor of hepatocellular carcinoma: A population based study. Hepatology 2012; 56: 241A.

[33] Mittal S, Sada YH, El-Serag HB, Kanwal F, Duan Z, Temple S, *et al.* Temporal trends of nonalcoholic Fatty liver disease-related hepatocellular carcinoma in the veteran affairs population. Clin Gastroenterol Hepatol 2015; 13: 594-601. e591
[http://dx.doi.org/10.1016/j.cgh.2014.08.013]

[34] Piscaglia F, Svegliati-Baroni G, Barchetti A, Pecorelli A, Marinelli S, Tiribelli C, *et al.* Clinical patterns of hepatocellular carcinoma (HCC) in non alcoholic fatty liver disease (NAFLD): A multicenter prospective study. Hepatology 2016; 63: 827-38.
[http://dx.doi.org/10.1016/S0168-8278(15)30554-7]

[35]   Ekstedt M, Franzén LE, Mathiesen UL, *et al.* Long-term follow-up of patients with NAFLD and elevated liver enzymes. Hepatology 2006; 44(4): 865-73.
[http://dx.doi.org/10.1002/hep.21327] [PMID: 17006923]

[36]   Rafiq N, Bai C, Fang Y, *et al.* Long-term follow-up of patients with nonalcoholic fatty liver. Clin Gastroenterol Hepatol 2009; 7(2): 234-8.
[http://dx.doi.org/10.1016/j.cgh.2008.11.005] [PMID: 19049831]

[37]   Chen CL, Yang HI, Yang WS, *et al.* Metabolic factors and risk of hepatocellular carcinoma by chronic hepatitis B/C infection: a follow-up study in Taiwan. Gastroenterology 2008; 135(1): 111-21.
[http://dx.doi.org/10.1053/j.gastro.2008.03.073] [PMID: 18505690]

[38]   Nair S, Mason A, Eason J, Loss G, Perrillo RP. Is obesity an independent risk factor for hepatocellular carcinoma in cirrhosis? Hepatology 2002; 36(1): 150-5.
[http://dx.doi.org/10.1053/jhep.2002.33713] [PMID: 12085359]

[39]   Pais R, Lebray P, Rousseau G, *et al.* Nonalcoholic fatty liver disease increases the risk of hepatocellular carcinoma in patients with alcohol-associated cirrhosis awaiting liver transplants. Clin Gastroenterol Hepatol 2015; 13(5): 992-9.e2.
[http://dx.doi.org/10.1016/j.cgh.2014.10.011] [PMID: 25459558]

[40]   Edenvik P, Davidsdottir L, Oksanen A, Isaksson B, Hultcrantz R, Stål P. Application of hepatocellular carcinoma surveillance in a European setting. What can we learn from clinical practice? Liver Int 2015; 35(7): 1862-71.
[http://dx.doi.org/10.1111/liv.12764] [PMID: 25524812]

[41]   Fattovich G, Stroffolini T, Zagni I, Donato F. Hepatocellular carcinoma in cirrhosis: incidence and risk factors. Gastroenterology 2004; 127(5) (Suppl. 1): S35-50.
[http://dx.doi.org/10.1053/j.gastro.2004.09.014] [PMID: 15508101]

[42]   Kondo Y, Kanai Y, Sakamoto M, Mizokami M, Ueda R, Hirohashi S. Genetic instability and aberrant DNA methylation in chronic hepatitis and cirrhosisA comprehensive study of loss of heterozygosity and microsatellite instability at 39 loci and DNA hypermethylation on 8 CpG islands in microdissected specimens from patients with hepatocellular carcinoma. Hepatology 2000; 32(5): 970-9.
[http://dx.doi.org/10.1053/jhep.2000.19797] [PMID: 11050047]

[43]   Aravalli RN, Cressman EN, Steer CJ. Cellular and molecular mechanisms of hepatocellular carcinoma: an update. Arch Toxicol 2013; 87(2): 227-47.
[http://dx.doi.org/10.1007/s00204-012-0931-2] [PMID: 23007558]

[44]   Zhang DY, Friedman SL. Fibrosis-dependent mechanisms of hepatocarcinogenesis. Hepatology 2012; 56(2): 769-75.
[http://dx.doi.org/10.1002/hep.25670] [PMID: 22378017]

[45]   Breuhahn K, Schirmacher P. Signaling networks in human hepatocarcinogenesisnovel aspects and therapeutic options. Prog Mol Biol Transl Sci 2010; 97: 251-77.
[http://dx.doi.org/10.1016/B978-0-12-385233-5.00009-X] [PMID: 21074736]

[46]   Thorgeirsson SS, Grisham JW. Molecular pathogenesis of human hepatocellular carcinoma. Nat Genet 2002; 31(4): 339-46.
[http://dx.doi.org/10.1038/ng0802-339] [PMID: 12149612]

[47]   Farazi PA, DePinho RA. Hepatocellular carcinoma pathogenesis: from genes to environment. Nat Rev Cancer 2006; 6(9): 674-87.
[http://dx.doi.org/10.1038/nrc1934] [PMID: 16929323]

[48]   Severi T, van Malenstein H, Verslype C, van Pelt JF. Tumor initiation and progression in hepatocellular carcinoma: risk factors, classification, and therapeutic targets. Acta Pharmacol Sin 2010; 31(11): 1409-20.

[49] Llovet JM, Chen Y, Wurmbach E, *et al.* A molecular signature to discriminate dysplastic nodules from early hepatocellular carcinoma in HCV cirrhosis. Gastroenterology 2006; 131(6): 1758-67.
[http://dx.doi.org/10.1053/j.gastro.2006.09.014] [PMID: 17087938]

[50] Breuhahn K, Longerich T, Schirmacher P. Dysregulation of growth factor signaling in human hepatocellular carcinoma. Oncogene 2006; 25(27): 3787-800.
[http://dx.doi.org/10.1038/sj.onc.1209556] [PMID: 16799620]

[51] Zhu AX. Molecularly targeted therapy for advanced hepatocellular carcinoma in 2012: current status and future perspectives. Semin Oncol 2012; 39(4): 493-502.
[http://dx.doi.org/10.1053/j.seminoncol.2012.05.014] [PMID: 22846866]

[52] Kitano H. Cancer as a robust system: implications for anticancer therapy. Nat Rev Cancer 2004; 4(3): 227-35.
[http://dx.doi.org/10.1038/nrc1300] [PMID: 14993904]

[53] Haslam DW, James WP. Obesity. Lancet 2005; 366(9492): 1197-209.
[http://dx.doi.org/10.1016/S0140-6736(05)67483-1] [PMID: 16198769]

[54] Hinney A, Hebebrand J. Polygenic obesity in humans. Obes Facts 2008; 1(1): 35-42.
[http://dx.doi.org/10.1159/000113935] [PMID: 20054160]

[55] Locke AE, Kahali B, Berndt SI, *et al.* Genetic studies of body mass index yield new insights for obesity biology. Nature 2015; 518(7538): 197-206.
[http://dx.doi.org/10.1038/nature14177] [PMID: 25673413]

[56] Shungin D, Winkler TW, Croteau-Chonka DC, *et al.* New genetic loci link adipose and insulin biology to body fat distribution. Nature 2015; 518(7538): 187-96.
[http://dx.doi.org/10.1038/nature14132] [PMID: 25673412]

[57] Anstee QM, Daly AK, Day CP. Genetics of alcoholic and nonalcoholic fatty liver disease. Semin Liver Dis 2011; 31(2): 128-46.
[http://dx.doi.org/10.1055/s-0031-1276643] [PMID: 21538280]

[58] Valenti L, Rumi M, Galmozzi E, *et al.* Patatin-like phospholipase domain-containing 3 I148M polymorphism, steatosis, and liver damage in chronic hepatitis C. Hepatology 2011; 53(3): 791-9.
[http://dx.doi.org/10.1002/hep.24123] [PMID: 21319195]

[59] Clarke JD, Novak P, Lake AD, *et al.* Characterization of hepatocellular carcinoma related genes and metabolites in human nonalcoholic fatty liver disease. Dig Dis Sci 2014; 59(2): 365-74.
[http://dx.doi.org/10.1007/s10620-013-2873-9] [PMID: 24048683]

[60] Leonardi GC, Candido S, Cervello M, *et al.* The tumor microenvironment in hepatocellular carcinoma (review). Int J Oncol 2012; 40(6): 1733-47. [review].
[PMID: 22447316]

[61] Starmann J, Fälth M, Spindelböck W, *et al.* Gene expression profiling unravels cancer-related hepatic molecular signatures in steatohepatitis but not in steatosis. PLoS One 2012; 7(10): e46584.
[http://dx.doi.org/10.1371/journal.pone.0046584] [PMID: 23071592]

[62] Anstee QM, Day CP. The Genetics of Nonalcoholic Fatty Liver Disease: Spotlight on PNPLA3 and TM6SF2. Semin Liver Dis 2015; 35(3): 270-90.
[http://dx.doi.org/10.1055/s-0035-1562947] [PMID: 26378644]

[63] Dongiovanni P, Petta S, Maglio C, *et al.* Transmembrane 6 superfamily member 2 gene variant disentangles nonalcoholic steatohepatitis from cardiovascular disease. Hepatology 2015; 61(2): 506-14.
[http://dx.doi.org/10.1002/hep.27490] [PMID: 25251399]

[64]   Smagris E, Gilyard S, BasuRay S, Cohen JC, Hobbs HH. Inactivation of Tm6sf2, a Gene Defective in Fatty Liver Disease, Impairs Lipidation but Not Secretion of Very Low Density Lipoproteins. J Biol Chem 2016; 291(20): 10659-76.
[http://dx.doi.org/10.1074/jbc.M116.719955] [PMID: 27013658]

[65]   Falleti E, Cussigh A, Cmet S, Fabris C, Toniutto P. PNPLA3 rs738409 and TM6SF2 rs58542926 variants increase the risk of hepatocellular carcinoma in alcoholic cirrhosis. Dig Liver Dis 2016; 48(1): 69-75.
[http://dx.doi.org/10.1016/j.dld.2015.09.009] [PMID: 26493626]

[66]   Shoelson SE, Herrero L, Naaz A. Obesity, inflammation, and insulin resistance. Gastroenterology 2007; 132(6): 2169-80.
[http://dx.doi.org/10.1053/j.gastro.2007.03.059] [PMID: 17498510]

[67]   Hotamisligil GS. Inflammation and metabolic disorders. Nature 2006; 444(7121): 860-7.
[http://dx.doi.org/10.1038/nature05485] [PMID: 17167474]

[68]   Marra F, Bertolani C. Adipokines in liver diseases. Hepatology 2009; 50(3): 957-69.
[http://dx.doi.org/10.1002/hep.23046] [PMID: 19585655]

[69]   Stickel F, Hellerbrand C. Non-alcoholic fatty liver disease as a risk factor for hepatocellular carcinoma: mechanisms and implications. Gut 2010; 59(10): 1303-7.
[http://dx.doi.org/10.1136/gut.2009.199661] [PMID: 20650925]

[70]   Karagozian R, Derdák Z, Baffy G. Obesity-associated mechanisms of hepatocarcinogenesis. Metabolism 2014; 63(5): 607-17.
[http://dx.doi.org/10.1016/j.metabol.2014.01.011] [PMID: 24629562]

[71]   Sun K, Kusminski CM, Scherer PE. Adipose tissue remodeling and obesity. J Clin Invest 2011; 121(6): 2094-101.
[http://dx.doi.org/10.1172/JCI45887] [PMID: 21633177]

[72]   He Q, Gao Z, Yin J, Zhang J, Yun Z, Ye J. Regulation of HIF-1alpha activity in adipose tissue by obesity-associated factors: adipogenesis, insulin, and hypoxia. Am J Physiol Endocrinol Metab 2011; 300(5): E877-85.
[http://dx.doi.org/10.1152/ajpendo.00626.2010] [PMID: 21343542]

[73]   Saxena NK, Sharma D, Ding X, *et al.* Concomitant activation of the JAK/STAT, PI3K/AKT, and ERK signaling is involved in leptin-mediated promotion of invasion and migration of hepatocellular carcinoma cells. Cancer Res 2007; 67(6): 2497-507.
[http://dx.doi.org/10.1158/0008-5472.CAN-06-3075] [PMID: 17363567]

[74]   Park EJ, Lee JH, Yu GY, *et al.* Dietary and genetic obesity promote liver inflammation and tumorigenesis by enhancing IL-6 and TNF expression. Cell 2010; 140(2): 197-208.
[http://dx.doi.org/10.1016/j.cell.2009.12.052] [PMID: 20141834]

[75]   Luo Z, Saha AK, Xiang X, Ruderman NB. AMPK, the metabolic syndrome and cancer. Trends Pharmacol Sci 2005; 26(2): 69-76.
[http://dx.doi.org/10.1016/j.tips.2004.12.011] [PMID: 15681023]

[76]   Browning JD, Horton JD. Molecular mediators of hepatic steatosis and liver injury. J Clin Invest 2004; 114(2): 147-52.
[http://dx.doi.org/10.1172/JCI200422422] [PMID: 15254578]

[77]   Postic C, Girard J. Contribution of de novo fatty acid synthesis to hepatic steatosis and insulin resistance: lessons from genetically engineered mice. J Clin Invest 2008; 118(3): 829-38.
[http://dx.doi.org/10.1172/JCI34275] [PMID: 18317565]

[78]   Pessayre D, Berson A, Fromenty B, Mansouri A. Mitochondria in steatohepatitis. Semin Liver Dis 2001; 21(1): 57-69.
        [http://dx.doi.org/10.1055/s-2001-12929] [PMID: 11296697]

[79]   Fujita K, Nozaki Y, Wada K, *et al.* Dysfunctional very-low-density lipoprotein synthesis and release is a key factor in nonalcoholic steatohepatitis pathogenesis. Hepatology 2009; 50(3): 772-80.
        [http://dx.doi.org/10.1002/hep.23094] [PMID: 19650159]

[80]   Shimomura I, Matsuda M, Hammer RE, Bashmakov Y, Brown MS, Goldstein JL. Decreased IRS-2 and increased SREBP-1c lead to mixed insulin resistance and sensitivity in livers of lipodystrophic and ob/ob mice. Mol Cell 2000; 6(1): 77-86.
        [http://dx.doi.org/10.1016/S1097-2765(05)00010-9] [PMID: 10949029]

[81]   Ferré P, Foufelle F. SREBP-1c transcription factor and lipid homeostasis: clinical perspective. Horm Res 2007; 68(2): 72-82.
        [PMID: 17344645]

[82]   Dalamaga M, Diakopoulos KN, Mantzoros CS. The role of adiponectin in cancer: a review of current evidence. Endocr Rev 2012; 33(4): 547-94.
        [http://dx.doi.org/10.1210/er.2011-1015] [PMID: 22547160]

[83]   Herman MA, Peroni OD, Villoria J, *et al.* A novel ChREBP isoform in adipose tissue regulates systemic glucose metabolism. Nature 2012; 484(7394): 333-8.
        [http://dx.doi.org/10.1038/nature10986] [PMID: 22466288]

[84]   Brown MS, Goldstein JL. Selective *versus* total insulin resistance: a pathogenic paradox. Cell Metab 2008; 7(2): 95-6.
        [http://dx.doi.org/10.1016/j.cmet.2007.12.009] [PMID: 18249166]

[85]   Lee JS, Mendez R, Heng HH, Yang ZQ, Zhang K. Pharmacological ER stress promotes hepatic lipogenesis and lipid droplet formation. Am J Transl Res 2012; 4(1): 102-13.
        [PMID: 22347525]

[86]   Unger RH, Orci L. Lipotoxic diseases of nonadipose tissues in obesity. Int J Obes Relat Metab Disord 2000; 24 (Suppl. 4): S28-32.
        [http://dx.doi.org/10.1038/sj.ijo.0801498] [PMID: 11126236]

[87]   Tan CY, Vidal-Puig A. Adipose tissue expandability: the metabolic problems of obesity may arise from the inability to become more obese. Biochem Soc Trans 2008; 36(Pt 5): 935-40.
        [http://dx.doi.org/10.1042/BST0360935] [PMID: 18793164]

[88]   Wu J, Kaufman RJ. From acute ER stress to physiological roles of the Unfolded Protein Response. Cell Death Differ 2006; 13(3): 374-84.
        [http://dx.doi.org/10.1038/sj.cdd.4401840] [PMID: 16397578]

[89]   Ozcan U, Cao Q, Yilmaz E, *et al.* Endoplasmic reticulum stress links obesity, insulin action, and type 2 diabetes. Science 2004; 306(5695): 457-61.
        [http://dx.doi.org/10.1126/science.1103160] [PMID: 15486293]

[90]   Hussain SP, Hofseth LJ, Harris CC. Radical causes of cancer. Nat Rev Cancer 2003; 3(4): 276-85.
        [http://dx.doi.org/10.1038/nrc1046] [PMID: 12671666]

[91]   Vinciguerra M, Carrozzino F, Peyrou M, *et al.* Unsaturated fatty acids promote hepatoma proliferation and progression through downregulation of the tumor suppressor PTEN. J Hepatol 2009; 50(6): 1132-41.
        [http://dx.doi.org/10.1016/j.jhep.2009.01.027] [PMID: 19398230]

[92]   Joshi-Barve S, Barve SS, Amancherla K, *et al.* Palmitic acid induces production of proinflammatory cytokine interleukin-8 from hepatocytes. Hepatology 2007; 46(3): 823-30.
        [http://dx.doi.org/10.1002/hep.21752] [PMID: 17680645]

[93] Baffy G. Kupffer cells in non-alcoholic fatty liver disease: the emerging view. J Hepatol 2009; 51(1): 212-23.
[http://dx.doi.org/10.1016/j.jhep.2009.03.008] [PMID: 19447517]

[94] Maeda S, Kamata H, Luo JL, Leffert H, Karin M. IKKbeta couples hepatocyte death to cytokine-driven compensatory proliferation that promotes chemical hepatocarcinogenesis. Cell 2005; 121(7): 977-90.
[http://dx.doi.org/10.1016/j.cell.2005.04.014] [PMID: 15989949]

[95] Sun B, Karin M. Obesity, inflammation, and liver cancer. J Hepatol 2012; 56(3): 704-13.
[http://dx.doi.org/10.1016/j.jhep.2011.09.020] [PMID: 22120206]

[96] Jiang S, Minter LC, Stratton SA, et al. TRIM24 suppresses development of spontaneous hepatic lipid accumulation and hepatocellular carcinoma in mice. J Hepatol 2015; 62(2): 371-9.
[http://dx.doi.org/10.1016/j.jhep.2014.09.026] [PMID: 25281858]

[97] Saltiel AR, Kahn CR. Insulin signalling and the regulation of glucose and lipid metabolism. Nature 2001; 414(6865): 799-806.
[http://dx.doi.org/10.1038/414799a] [PMID: 11742412]

[98] Khandekar MJ, Cohen P, Spiegelman BM. Molecular mechanisms of cancer development in obesity. Nat Rev Cancer 2011; 11(12): 886-95.
[http://dx.doi.org/10.1038/nrc3174] [PMID: 22113164]

[99] Kim KW, Bae SK, Lee OH, Bae MH, Lee MJ, Park BC. Insulin-like growth factor II induced by hypoxia may contribute to angiogenesis of human hepatocellular carcinoma. Cancer Res 1998; 58(2): 348-51.
[PMID: 9443416]

[100] Tanaka S, Mohr L, Schmidt EV, Sugimachi K, Wands JR. Biological effects of human insulin receptor substrate-1 overexpression in hepatocytes. Hepatology 1997; 26(3): 598-604.
[http://dx.doi.org/10.1002/hep.510260310] [PMID: 9303488]

[101] De Minicis S, Agostinelli L, Rychlicki C, et al. HCC development is associated to peripheral insulin resistance in a mouse model of NASH. PLoS One 2014; 9(5): e97136.
[http://dx.doi.org/10.1371/journal.pone.0097136] [PMID: 24853141]

[102] Schwabe RF, Jobin C. The microbiome and cancer. Nat Rev Cancer 2013; 13(11): 800-12.
[http://dx.doi.org/10.1038/nrc3610] [PMID: 24132111]

[103] Tilg H, Kaser A. Gut microbiome, obesity, and metabolic dysfunction. J Clin Invest 2011; 121(6): 2126-32.
[http://dx.doi.org/10.1172/JCI58109] [PMID: 21633181]

[104] Zhao L. The gut microbiota and obesity: from correlation to causality. Nat Rev Microbiol 2013; 11(9): 639-47.
[http://dx.doi.org/10.1038/nrmicro3089] [PMID: 23912213]

[105] Schuppan D, Afdhal NH. Liver cirrhosis. Lancet 2008; 371(9615): 838-51.
[http://dx.doi.org/10.1016/S0140-6736(08)60383-9] [PMID: 18328931]

[106] Szabo G, Dolganiuc A, Mandrekar P. Pattern recognition receptors: a contemporary view on liver diseases. Hepatology 2006; 44(2): 287-98.
[http://dx.doi.org/10.1002/hep.21308] [PMID: 16871558]

[107] Dapito DH, Mencin A, Gwak GY, et al. Promotion of hepatocellular carcinoma by the intestinal microbiota and TLR4. Cancer Cell 2012; 21(4): 504-16.
[http://dx.doi.org/10.1016/j.ccr.2012.02.007] [PMID: 22516259]

[108]   Yoshimoto S, Loo TM, Atarashi K, *et al.* Obesity-induced gut microbial metabolite promotes liver cancer through senescence secretome. Nature 2013; 499(7456): 97-101.
[http://dx.doi.org/10.1038/nature12347] [PMID: 23803760]

[109]   Bartel DP. MicroRNAs: genomics, biogenesis, mechanism, and function. Cell 2004; 116(2): 281-97.
[http://dx.doi.org/10.1016/S0092-8674(04)00045-5] [PMID: 14744438]

[110]   Moore KJ, Rayner KJ, Suárez Y, Fernández-Hernando C. The role of microRNAs in cholesterol efflux and hepatic lipid metabolism. Annu Rev Nutr 2011; 31: 49-63.
[http://dx.doi.org/10.1146/annurev-nutr-081810-160756] [PMID: 21548778]

[111]   Lu J, Getz G, Miska EA, *et al.* MicroRNA expression profiles classify human cancers. Nature 2005; 435(7043): 834-8.
[http://dx.doi.org/10.1038/nature03702] [PMID: 15944708]

[112]   Mott JL. MicroRNAs involved in tumor suppressor and oncogene pathways: implications for hepatobiliary neoplasia. Hepatology 2009; 50(2): 630-7.
[http://dx.doi.org/10.1002/hep.23010] [PMID: 19585622]

[113]   Huang S, He X. The role of microRNAs in liver cancer progression. Br J Cancer 2011; 104(2): 235-40.
[http://dx.doi.org/10.1038/sj.bjc.6606010] [PMID: 21102580]

[114]   Augello C, Vaira V, Caruso L, *et al.* MicroRNA profiling of hepatocarcinogenesis identifies C19MC cluster as a novel prognostic biomarker in hepatocellular carcinoma. Liver Int 2012; 32(5): 772-82.
[http://dx.doi.org/10.1111/j.1478-3231.2012.02795.x] [PMID: 22429613]

[115]   Fukuhara T, Matsuura Y. Role of miR-122 and lipid metabolism in HCV infection. J Gastroenterol 2013; 48(2): 169-76.
[http://dx.doi.org/10.1007/s00535-012-0661-5] [PMID: 22965312]

[116]   Takaki Y, Saito Y, Takasugi A, *et al.* Silencing of microRNA-122 is an early event during hepatocarcinogenesis from non-alcoholic steatohepatitis. Cancer Sci 2014; 105(10): 1254-60.
[http://dx.doi.org/10.1111/cas.12498] [PMID: 25117675]

[117]   Rottiers V, Näär AM. MicroRNAs in metabolism and metabolic disorders. Nat Rev Mol Cell Biol 2012; 13(4): 239-50.
[http://dx.doi.org/10.1038/nrm3313] [PMID: 22436747]

[118]   Cheung O, Puri P, Eicken C, *et al.* Nonalcoholic steatohepatitis is associated with altered hepatic MicroRNA expression. Hepatology 2008; 48(6): 1810-20.
[http://dx.doi.org/10.1002/hep.22569] [PMID: 19030170]

[119]   Derdak Z, Villegas KA, Harb R, Wu AM, Sousa A, Wands JR. Inhibition of p53 attenuates steatosis and liver injury in a mouse model of non-alcoholic fatty liver disease. J Hepatol 2013; 58(4): 785-91.
[http://dx.doi.org/10.1016/j.jhep.2012.11.042] [PMID: 23211317]

[120]   Hermeking H. p53 enters the microRNA world. Cancer Cell 2007; 12(5): 414-8.
[http://dx.doi.org/10.1016/j.ccr.2007.10.028] [PMID: 17996645]

[121]   Tornesello ML, Buonaguro L, Tatangelo F, Botti G, Izzo F, Buonaguro FM. Mutations in TP53, CTNNB1 and PIK3CA genes in hepatocellular carcinoma associated with hepatitis B and hepatitis C virus infections. Genomics 2013; 102(2): 74-83.
[http://dx.doi.org/10.1016/j.ygeno.2013.04.001] [PMID: 23583669]

[122]   Wu H, Ng R, Chen X, Steer CJ, Song G. MicroRNA-21 is a potential link between non-alcoholic fatty liver disease and hepatocellular carcinoma *via* modulation of the HBP1-p53-Srebp1c pathway. Gut 2015; •••: gutjnl-2014-308430.
[http://dx.doi.org/10.1136/gutjnl-2014-308430] [PMID: 26282675]

[123] Cermelli S, Ruggieri A, Marrero JA, Ioannou GN, Beretta L. Circulating microRNAs in patients with chronic hepatitis C and non-alcoholic fatty liver disease. PLoS One 2011; 6(8): e23937.
[http://dx.doi.org/10.1371/journal.pone.0023937] [PMID: 21886843]

[124] Sacco J, Adeli K. MicroRNAs: emerging roles in lipid and lipoprotein metabolism. Curr Opin Lipidol 2012; 23(3): 220-5.
[http://dx.doi.org/10.1097/MOL.0b013e3283534c9f] [PMID: 22488426]

[125] Estep M, Armistead D, Hossain N, *et al.* Differential expression of miRNAs in the visceral adipose tissue of patients with non-alcoholic fatty liver disease. Aliment Pharmacol Ther 2010; 32(3): 487-97.
[http://dx.doi.org/10.1111/j.1365-2036.2010.04366.x] [PMID: 20497147]

[126] Jiang J, Gusev Y, Aderca I, *et al.* Association of MicroRNA expression in hepatocellular carcinomas with hepatitis infection, cirrhosis, and patient survival. Clin Cancer Res 2008; 14(2): 419-27.
[http://dx.doi.org/10.1158/1078-0432.CCR-07-0523] [PMID: 18223217]

[127] Gori M, Arciello M, Balsano C. MicroRNAs in nonalcoholic fatty liver disease: novel biomarkers and prognostic tools during the transition from steatosis to hepatocarcinoma. Biomed Res Int 2014; 2014: 741465.
[http://dx.doi.org/10.1155/2014/741465]

[128] Paradis V, Zalinski S, Chelbi E, *et al.* Hepatocellular carcinomas in patients with metabolic syndrome often develop without significant liver fibrosis: a pathological analysis. Hepatology 2009; 49(3): 851-9.
[http://dx.doi.org/10.1002/hep.22734] [PMID: 19115377]

[129] Brancatelli G, Federle MP, Grazioli L, Carr BI. Hepatocellular carcinoma in noncirrhotic liver: CT, clinical, and pathologic findings in 39 U.S. residents. Radiology 2002; 222(1): 89-94.
[http://dx.doi.org/10.1148/radiol.2221010767] [PMID: 11756710]

[130] Bugianesi E, Leone N, Vanni E, *et al.* Expanding the natural history of nonalcoholic steatohepatitis: from cryptogenic cirrhosis to hepatocellular carcinoma. Gastroenterology 2002; 123(1): 134-40.
[http://dx.doi.org/10.1053/gast.2002.34168] [PMID: 12105842]

[131] Regimbeau JM, Colombat M, Mognol P, *et al.* Obesity and diabetes as a risk factor for hepatocellular carcinoma. Liver Transpl 2004; 10(2) (Suppl. 1): S69-73.
[http://dx.doi.org/10.1002/lt.20033] [PMID: 14762843]

[132] Kawada N, Imanaka K, Kawaguchi T, *et al.* Hepatocellular carcinoma arising from non-cirrhotic nonalcoholic steatohepatitis. J Gastroenterol 2009; 44(12): 1190-4.
[http://dx.doi.org/10.1007/s00535-009-0112-0] [PMID: 19672551]

[133] Yasui K, Hashimoto E, Komorizono Y, *et al.* Characteristics of patients with nonalcoholic steatohepatitis who develop hepatocellular carcinoma. Clin Gastroenterol Hepatol 2011; 9(5): 428-33.
[http://dx.doi.org/10.1016/j.cgh.2011.01.023] [PMID: 21320639]

[134] Iannaccone R, Piacentini F, Murakami T, *et al.* Hepatocellular carcinoma in patients with nonalcoholic fatty liver disease: helical CT and MR imaging findings with clinical-pathologic comparison. Radiology 2007; 243(2): 422-30.
[http://dx.doi.org/10.1148/radiol.2432051244] [PMID: 17356175]

[135] Leung C, Yeoh SW, Patrick D, *et al.* Characteristics of hepatocellular carcinoma in cirrhotic and non-cirrhotic non-alcoholic fatty liver disease. World J Gastroenterol 2015; 21(4): 1189-96.
[http://dx.doi.org/10.3748/wjg.v21.i4.1189] [PMID: 25632192]

[136] Marrero JA, Su GL, Wei W, *et al.* Des-gamma carboxyprothrombin can differentiate hepatocellular carcinoma from nonmalignant chronic liver disease in American patients. Hepatology 2003; 37(5): 1114-21.
[http://dx.doi.org/10.1053/jhep.2003.50195] [PMID: 12717392]

[137]   Oka H, Tamori A, Kuroki T, Kobayashi K, Yamamoto S. Prospective study of alpha-fetoprotein in cirrhotic patients monitored for development of hepatocellular carcinoma. Hepatology 1994; 19(1): 61-6.
[http://dx.doi.org/10.1002/hep.1840190111] [PMID: 7506227]

[138]   Voiculescu M, Nanau RM, Neuman MG. Non-invasive biomarkers in non-alcoholic steatohepatitis-induced hepatocellular carcinoma. J Gastrointestin Liver Dis 2014; 23(4): 425-9.
[PMID: 25532002]

[139]   Davila JA, Morgan RO, Richardson PA, Du XL, McGlynn KA, El-Serag HB. Use of surveillance for hepatocellular carcinoma among patients with cirrhosis in the United States. Hepatology 2010; 52(1): 132-41.
[http://dx.doi.org/10.1002/hep.23615] [PMID: 20578139]

[140]   Gupta S, Bent S, Kohlwes J. Test characteristics of alpha-fetoprotein for detecting hepatocellular carcinoma in patients with hepatitis C. A systematic review and critical analysis. Ann Intern Med 2003; 139(1): 46-50.
[http://dx.doi.org/10.7326/0003-4819-139-1-200307010-00012] [PMID: 12834318]

[141]   Sherman M. Surveillance for hepatocellular carcinoma. Semin Oncol 2001; 28(5): 450-9.
[http://dx.doi.org/10.1016/S0093-7754(01)90138-1] [PMID: 11685738]

[142]   Miao R, Luo H, Zhou H, *et al.* Identification of prognostic biomarkers in hepatitis B virus-related hepatocellular carcinoma and stratification by integrative multi-omics analysis. J Hepatol 2014; 61(4): 840-9.
[http://dx.doi.org/10.1016/j.jhep.2014.05.025] [PMID: 24859455]

[143]   Jin GZ, Li Y, Cong WM, *et al.* iTRAQ-2DLC-ESI-MS/MS based identification of a new set of immunohistochemical biomarkers for classification of dysplastic nodules and small hepatocellular carcinoma. J Proteome Res 2011; 10(8): 3418-28.
[http://dx.doi.org/10.1021/pr200482t] [PMID: 21631109]

[144]   Nishida N, Kudo M, Nishimura T, *et al.* Unique association between global DNA hypomethylation and chromosomal alterations in human hepatocellular carcinoma. PLoS One 2013; 8(9): e72312.
[http://dx.doi.org/10.1371/journal.pone.0072312] [PMID: 24023736]

[145]   Baffy G. The impact of network medicine in gastroenterology and hepatology. Clin Gastroenterol Hepatol 2013; 11(10): 1240-4.
[http://dx.doi.org/10.1016/j.cgh.2013.07.033] [PMID: 23932906]

[146]   Torres DM, Harrison SA. Nonalcoholic steatohepatitis and noncirrhotic hepatocellular carcinoma: fertile soil. Semin Liver Dis 2012; 32(1): 30-8.
[http://dx.doi.org/10.1055/s-0032-1306424] [PMID: 22418886]

[147]   Caldwell SH, Oelsner DH, Iezzoni JC, Hespenheide EE, Battle EH, Driscoll CJ. Cryptogenic cirrhosis: clinical characterization and risk factors for underlying disease. Hepatology 1999; 29(3): 664-9.
[http://dx.doi.org/10.1002/hep.510290347] [PMID: 10051466]

[148]   Poonawala A, Nair SP, Thuluvath PJ. Prevalence of obesity and diabetes in patients with cryptogenic cirrhosis: a case-control study. Hepatology 2000; 32(4 Pt 1): 689-92.
[http://dx.doi.org/10.1053/jhep.2000.17894] [PMID: 11003611]

[149]   Marrero JA, Fontana RJ, Su GL, Conjeevaram HS, Emick DM, Lok AS. NAFLD may be a common underlying liver disease in patients with hepatocellular carcinoma in the United States. Hepatology 2002; 36(6): 1349-54.
[http://dx.doi.org/10.1002/hep.1840360609] [PMID: 12447858]

[150] Cortez-Pinto H, Jesus L, Barros H, Lopes C, Moura MC, Camilo ME. How different is the dietary pattern in non-alcoholic steatohepatitis patients? Clin Nutr 2006; 25(5): 816-23.
[http://dx.doi.org/10.1016/j.clnu.2006.01.027] [PMID: 16677739]

[151] Church TS, Kuk JL, Ross R, Priest EL, Biltoft E, Blair SN. Association of cardiorespiratory fitness, body mass index, and waist circumference to nonalcoholic fatty liver disease. Gastroenterology 2006; 130(7): 2023-30.
[http://dx.doi.org/10.1053/j.gastro.2006.03.019] [PMID: 16762625]

[152] Adams TD, Gress RE, Smith SC, *et al.* Long-term mortality after gastric bypass surgery. N Engl J Med 2007; 357(8): 753-61.
[http://dx.doi.org/10.1056/NEJMoa066603] [PMID: 17715409]

[153] Sjöström L. Review of the key results from the Swedish Obese Subjects (SOS) trial - a prospective controlled intervention study of bariatric surgery. J Intern Med 2013; 273(3): 219-34.
[http://dx.doi.org/10.1111/joim.12012] [PMID: 23163728]

[154] Piguet AC, Saran U, Simillion C, *et al.* Regular exercise decreases liver tumors development in hepatocyte-specific PTEN-deficient mice independently of steatosis. J Hepatol 2015; 62(6): 1296-303.
[http://dx.doi.org/10.1016/j.jhep.2015.01.017] [PMID: 25623824]

[155] Yang Y, Zhang D, Feng N, *et al.* Increased intake of vegetables, but not fruit, reduces risk for hepatocellular carcinoma: a meta-analysis. Gastroenterology 2014; 147(5): 1031-42.
[http://dx.doi.org/10.1053/j.gastro.2014.08.005] [PMID: 25127680]

[156] Donadon V, Balbi M, Mas MD, Casarin P, Zanette G. Metformin and reduced risk of hepatocellular carcinoma in diabetic patients with chronic liver disease. Liver Int 2010; 30(5): 750-8.
[http://dx.doi.org/10.1111/j.1478-3231.2010.02223.x] [PMID: 20331505]

[157] Chen HP, Shieh JJ, Chang CC, *et al.* Metformin decreases hepatocellular carcinoma risk in a dose-dependent manner: population-based and *in vitro* studies. Gut 2013; 62(4): 606-15.
[http://dx.doi.org/10.1136/gutjnl-2011-301708] [PMID: 22773548]

[158] Kilaru S, Baffy G. Metformin and hepatocellular carcinoma. J Sympt Signs 2015; 4: 15-24.

[159] Hassan MM, Curley SA, Li D, *et al.* Association of diabetes duration and diabetes treatment with the risk of hepatocellular carcinoma. Cancer 2010; 116(8): 1938-46.
[http://dx.doi.org/10.1002/cncr.24982] [PMID: 20166205]

[160] Aljada A, Mousa SA. Metformin and neoplasia: implications and indications. Pharmacol Ther 2012; 133(1): 108-15.
[http://dx.doi.org/10.1016/j.pharmthera.2011.09.004] [PMID: 21924289]

[161] Bhalla K, Hwang BJ, Dewi RE, *et al.* Metformin prevents liver tumorigenesis by inhibiting pathways driving hepatic lipogenesis. Cancer Prev Res (Phila) 2012; 5(4): 544-52.
[http://dx.doi.org/10.1158/1940-6207.CAPR-11-0228] [PMID: 22467080]

[162] Batandier C, Guigas B, Detaille D, *et al.* The ROS production induced by a reverse-electron flux at respiratory-chain complex 1 is hampered by metformin. J Bioenerg Biomembr 2006; 38(1): 33-42.
[http://dx.doi.org/10.1007/s10863-006-9003-8] [PMID: 16732470]

[163] Haukeland JW, Konopski Z, Eggesbø HB, *et al.* Metformin in patients with non-alcoholic fatty liver disease: a randomized, controlled trial. Scand J Gastroenterol 2009; 44(7): 853-60.
[http://dx.doi.org/10.1080/00365520902845268] [PMID: 19811343]

[164] Lavine JE, Schwimmer JB, Van Natta ML, *et al.* Effect of vitamin E or metformin for treatment of nonalcoholic fatty liver disease in children and adolescents: the TONIC randomized controlled trial. JAMA 2011; 305(16): 1659-68.
[http://dx.doi.org/10.1001/jama.2011.520] [PMID: 21521847]

[165] Singh S, Singh PP, Singh AG, Murad MH, Sanchez W. Statins are associated with a reduced risk of hepatocellular cancer: a systematic review and meta-analysis. Gastroenterology 2013; 144(2): 323-32.
[http://dx.doi.org/10.1053/j.gastro.2012.10.005] [PMID: 23063971]

[166] McGlynn KA, Divine GW, Sahasrabuddhe VV, *et al.* Statin use and risk of hepatocellular carcinoma in a U.S. population. Cancer Epidemiol 2014; 38(5): 523-7.
[http://dx.doi.org/10.1016/j.canep.2014.06.009] [PMID: 25113938]

[167] Jeon CY, Goodman MT, Cook-Wiens G, Sundaram V. Statin Use and Survival with Early-Stage Hepatocellular Carcinoma. Cancer Epidemiol Biomarkers Prev 2016; 25(4): 686-92.
[http://dx.doi.org/10.1158/1055-9965.EPI-15-1040] [PMID: 26908429]

[168] Wang YD, Chen WD, Moore DD, Huang W. FXR: a metabolic regulator and cell protector. Cell Res 2008; 18(11): 1087-95.
[http://dx.doi.org/10.1038/cr.2008.289] [PMID: 18825165]

[169] Kaul S, Rothney MP, Peters DM, *et al.* Dual-energy X-ray absorptiometry for quantification of visceral fat. Obesity (Silver Spring) 2012; 20(6): 1313-8.
[http://dx.doi.org/10.1038/oby.2011.393] [PMID: 22282048]

[170] Huang W, Ma K, Zhang J, *et al.* Nuclear receptor-dependent bile acid signaling is required for normal liver regeneration. Science 2006; 312(5771): 233-6.
[http://dx.doi.org/10.1126/science.1121435] [PMID: 16614213]

[171] Modica S, Murzilli S, Salvatore L, Schmidt DR, Moschetta A. Nuclear bile acid receptor FXR protects against intestinal tumorigenesis. Cancer Res 2008; 68(23): 9589-94.
[http://dx.doi.org/10.1158/0008-5472.CAN-08-1791] [PMID: 19047134]

[172] Deuschle U, Schüler J, Schulz A, *et al.* FXR controls the tumor suppressor NDRG2 and FXR agonists reduce liver tumor growth and metastasis in an orthotopic mouse xenograft model. PLoS One 2012; 7(10): e43044.
[http://dx.doi.org/10.1371/journal.pone.0043044] [PMID: 23056173]

[173] Wolfe A, Thomas A, Edwards G, Jaseja R, Guo GL, Apte U. Increased activation of the Wnt/β-catenin pathway in spontaneous hepatocellular carcinoma observed in farnesoid X receptor knockout mice. J Pharmacol Exp Ther 2011; 338(1): 12-21.
[http://dx.doi.org/10.1124/jpet.111.179390] [PMID: 21430080]

[174] Jiang Y, Iakova P, Jin J, *et al.* Farnesoid X receptor inhibits gankyrin in mouse livers and prevents development of liver cancer. Hepatology 2013; 57(3): 1098-106.
[http://dx.doi.org/10.1002/hep.26146] [PMID: 23172628]

[175] Neuschwander-Tetri BA, Loomba R, Sanyal AJ, *et al.* Farnesoid X nuclear receptor ligand obeticholic acid for non-cirrhotic, non-alcoholic steatohepatitis (FLINT): a multicentre, randomised, placebo-controlled trial. Lancet 2015; 385(9972): 956-65.
[http://dx.doi.org/10.1016/S0140-6736(14)61933-4] [PMID: 25468160]

CHAPTER 9

Non-Alcoholic Fatty Liver Disease in the Pediatric Population

Zsuzsanna Almássy[*]

Department of Toxicology and Metabolic Diseases, Heim Pál Children's Hospital, Budapest, Hungary

Abstract: In the past decade, obesity has reached epidemic magnitude among children and adolescents, thus associated pathologic conditions are increasing simultaneously. These conditions include insulin resistance, type 2 diabetes, metabolic syndrome, cardiovascular diseases (CVD) and fatty liver disease (NAFLD).

NAFLD, previously thought to impact adults only, shares many of the same features of the metabolic syndrome, a highly atherogenic condition. This drew increased focus to study the role of NAFLD in relation to higher overall mortality and morbidity rates and increased prevalence of cardiovascular disease (CVD).

Insulin resistance is the pathophysiologic hallmark of NAFLD, the most common form of chronic liver disease in children in today's time. It is characterized by triglyceride accumulation with secondary free-radical production, which induces inflammatory processes and fibrosis due to numerous causes and complex mechanism.

Recent studies indicate that NAFLD has high prevalence in obese children, which has serious cosequences without treatment. Early intervention is utmost important when NAFLD is diagnosed, which should include early lifestyle modification (nutrition and physical activity, avoidance of smoking), however, no evidence based therapeutic approaches exist.

Keywords: Cardiovascular risk, Children, Insulin resistance, Nonalcoholic fatty liver disease, Obesity.

INTRODUCTION

Being obese or overweight in childhood increases the risk of being overweight or obese in later life. Similar to adult obesity, childhood obesity has been associated with a number of comorbidities [1].

[*] **Corresponding author Zsuzsanna Almássy:** Department of Toxicology and Metabolic Diseases, Heim Pál Children's Hospital, Budapest, 1089 Budapest, Üllői út 86, Hungary; E-mail: almassy.zsuzsa@t-online.hu

Tatjana Ábel & Gabriella Lengyel (Eds.)
All rights reserved-© 2017 Bentham Science Publishers

As obesity is a growing epidemy throughout the world, including Hungary, where nearly one third of children between the age of 6-12 years are overweight or obese, problems rising from this condition are becoming a great burden for the individual and for the society as well. A number of associated conditions, like metabolic syndrome, cardiovascular disease, type 2 diabetes (T2DM), fatty liver are observed already in childhood. Fatty liver is presently the most common liver disease in children [2, 3, 35].

Liver plays a key role in glucose homeostasis, as it receives and metabolizes the absorbed nutrients, stores or redistributes them according to the actual metabolic state of the person. It is important to understand that glucose metabolism is highly dependent on liver function, and the liver also plays an important role in the metabolism of drugs, produces inflammatory and vasoactive factors. Glucose overload increases fat accumulation in the liver.

By definition, nonalcoholic fatty liver disease (NAFLD) is the accumulation of triglyceride in the liver in more than 5% of hepatocytes with a reported prevalence of 3% to 10% in the general pediatric population and reaching a prevalence of 80% in obese/overweight children [4]. NAFLD can also be described as the metabolic disease of the liver [5], which can be seen quite early in children.

A number of causes can be found in the development of NAFLD, the leading cause being central obesity in childhood with insulin resistance, which in turn is the consequence of high-energy intake food and sedentary lifestyle. These associations are partly mediated by fat mass and fat quality.

EPIDEMIOLOGY, PATHOGENESIS

The realistic prevalence of NAFLD in the general population is estimated to be around 30%, even with the widely varying epidemiological data [6]. The prevalence rises further in adults with obesity (57-98%) and diabetes (69%) reflecting the strong association with metabolic syndrome [7, 8]. A life-cycle analysis showed a reduction of life expectancy with up to 7 years in adults with obesity [9].

It is estimated that 170 million children under 18 years old worldwide are overweight or obese, which is more than 20% of all children in many countries [15].

Insulin resistance is often accompanied by NAFLD/NASH, and plays a leading role in its pathophysiology [10, 11].

Those who had altered liver function as well, namely elevated ALT were shown to have a threefold risk for developing type 2 diabetes (T2DM) in a study, but the correlation disappeared after the multivariate regression analysis in one study, so authors stated that NAFLD was not an independent predictor [12]. Nevertheless in other studies, authors found that NAFLD was an independent predictor of T2DM and a strong risk factor for prediabetes [13, 14].

Comorbidities, as fatty liver is increased in this population. According to the follow-up study by Feldstein *et al.*, 4 out of the 66 children with NAFLD develop T2DM 4-11 years after the diagnosis. Moreover, during a 20-year long follow-up study, 2 children died and 2 underwent liver transplantation for cirrhosis, though formerly childhood fatty liver was considered a benign alteration [16]. Nevertheless there are only sporadic data regarding children till now.

Fatty liver classification is based on the severity of the liver status from simple steatosis (NAFLD) to steatosis with fibrosis, necrosis and inflammation (NASH). In the last year, alarming reports have been published about NAFLD in childhood, for this population tends to be overweight and obese due to excess food intake and sedentary lifestyle [17, 18]. NAFLD is often described as the metabolic syndrome of the liver that may start early in life with a generational transfer from mothers with high BMI to their offsprings [19]. Thus NAFLD is strongly associated not only with metabolic syndrome and type 2 diabetes, but also with cardiovascular disease. Prediabetes was reported to reach 85% in NAFLD patients [5].

Though the complete pathogenesis remains still unexplained and differs from adults, insulin resistance seems to be the main background, with other pathological conditions involved.

NAFLD is often described as a two-hit or multiple-hit model, where the first-hit involves triglyceride (TG) accumulation in hepatocytes exceeding 5% of cells, and liver damage as second -hit, or further hits, depending on the origin and extent of damage (fibrosis). That has been accepted in adults, however in children fibrosis did not correlate with insulin resistance. In children, the second phase is more variable and most often reversible. Fibrosis rarely occurs, even if it does, however, it does not correlate with insulin resistance. Genetic predisposition and environmental factors are the possible factors to act as second-hits in children.

Heterogenous genetic background also contributes to the evolution of children's fatty liver disease, *e.g.* chromosomal abnormalities, as Turner syndrome, Down syndrome, inherited metabolic syndromes (Prader-Willi, Angelman, Bardet-Biedl, Cohen, *etc.*), inherited metabolic diseases, like mitochondrial and fatty acid metabolic diseases, and some other conditions, *eg*: nephrotic syndrome [20, 39].

Environmental factors can also generate fatty alteration of the liver, like some hormonal therapies (steroids), total parenteral nutrition, maternal weight gain during pregnancy, pre-pregnancy parental BMI with stronger association with maternal BMI are also predisposing factors [21, 22].

Oxidative stress, endotoxins, adipocytokines /TNF-alfa, adiponectin, leptin/ are considered as hepatocyte damaging factors of the second hit [23]. Hypoxia caused by sleep apnea is a frequent finding is obese children, which also has a negative effect as well.

Nowadays, great attention is paid to the gut-liver axis malfunction causing small intestinal bacterial overgrowth, intestinal dysbiosis, increased intestinal permeability (leaky gut), also considered as an important factor leading to the development and progression of NAFLD [8].

The basic pathology is the riglyceride triglyceride storage in hepatocytes. In the onset and progression of obesity, associated with insulin resistance, increased free fatty acid levels and abnormal adipocytokine secretion are important factors.

Deposition of riglyceride triglyceride (TG) in hepatocytes is determined by the balance of TG- increasing factors (influx and synthesis of TG) and TG-decreasing factors (efflux and consumption). Triglyceride is composed of 3 fatty acids esterified to a glycerol. Four mechanisms are suspected to affect hepatocytes' TGs level:

1. Increased uptake of free fatty acids (FFA) from food and fatty tissue that accounts for the FFA pool in the blood.
2. Increased *de novo* FFA synthesis in liver cells, or reduction of the suppression of FFA synthesis.
3. Decreased catabolism of FFA in liver cells (consumption by poxisomes and mitochondrial beta-oxidation).
4. Decreased release of TG from hepatocytes (very-low-density lipoprotein is released into the blood by microsomal triglyceride protein) [23, 24].

Histologically NAFLD is divided into two categories: sample steatosis and fibrosis with necrosis and inflammation, called nonalcoholic steatohepatitis (NASH).

Nonalcoholic steatohepatitis (NASH) in children was described by Moran and coworkers in 1983, so the term is well known since then [25].

This clinical entity is defined by clinical symptoms, laboratory alterations, and clinical imaging (Fig. **1**).

NAFLD AND CVD IN CHILDREN

Several studies performed in the pediatric population revealed that the rising prevalence of obesity-related metabolic syndrome and NAFLD in childhood may lead to a parallel increase in adverse cardiovascular outcomes. In children, cardiovascular system's damage is reversible if early interventions are introduced timely and effectively.

In the cohort of children, the earliest clinical sign of macrovascular changes is elevated systolic blood pressure, which if treated at appropriate time can be reversed entirely.

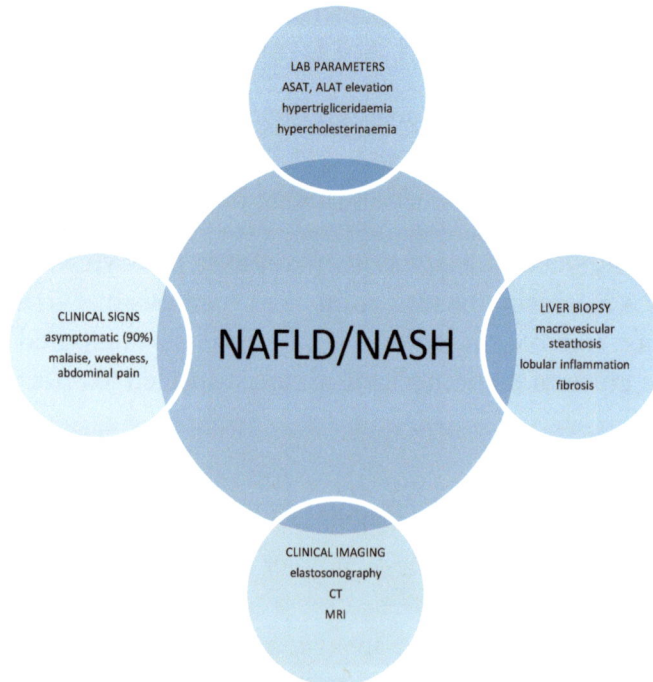

Fig. (1). The basis of alterations.

Many adolescents with NAFLD already have subclinical atherosclerosis. The growing evidence from several studies strongly emphasizes the importance of evaluating the CVD risk in pediatric NAFLD [26, 27].

Jin and coworkers evaluated the volume of intrahepatic fat in a cohort of hispanic-american overweight adolescents and found that higher accumulation of liver fat has strong association with peripheral atherogenic dyslipidaemia, namely higher triglyceride levels, and higher TG/HDL rate. The above findings suggest that hepatic fat (NAFLD) is not only a marker of CVD risk, but also an important mediator in the pathogenesis of subclinical, early atherosclerosis independent of insulin resistance [28].

Greater overall energy intake increases total body fat, thus elevating the risk of fat infiltration into the liver, causing disequilibrium in the rate of TG/HDL levels. Overproduction of TG rich lipoprotein (TRL) activates the enzyme cholesterol ester transfer protein (CETP) leading to an increase in the exchange of cholesterol ester and triglyceride between the TRL and LDL. This transfer protein mediated interaction produces substrates for further lipolysis and clearance by hepatic lipase, promoting the formation of small dense LDL. It is well established that small LDL has low affinity to LDL receptors and is more susceptible to oxidative modification, which in turn predisposes atherogenic alterations in blood vessels [28 - 30].

On one hand it is postulated that hyperinsulinemia and insulin resistance are key metabolic defects resulting in increased accumulation of hepatocellular triglyceride. On the other hand, it is also possible that primary dysregulation of lipoprotein metabolism, including overproduction and impaired secretion of hepatic triglycerides contributes to hepatic steatosis independent of insulin resistance [31, 32]. A large-scale multi-ethnic study in adults also indicated strong correlation between NAFLD with atherogenic dyslipidemia phenotype in a dose dependent way [33].

This dose effect was observed by others in a pediatric cohort as well, stating that an increased volume of hepatic fat was strongly associated with a more atherogenic lipid profile independent of insulin resistance, including increased concentration of large VLDL, greater size of VLDL particles, elevated small dense LDL particles [28]. This might explain early manifestations of subclinical atherosclerosis in adolescents with NAFLD. Whether reduction of hepatic fat is reducing cardiovascular risk in NAFLD on the long run, still needs to be studied.

RISK AND DEVELOPMENT OF NAFLD

Obesity is the major risk factor of fatty liver in childhood. A number of studies found a threefold increase of NAFLD in obese children, the prevalence being 9.6% in healthy- and 28% in obese children [34]. In Hungary, every 4th child is overweight or obese, so there are a great number of children with undiagnosed NAFLD just like in the UK [35]. Other common risk factors include genetically determined and environmental factors, listed in Table **1**.

DEVELOPMENT OF NAFLD

NAFLD is a multifactorial condition as seen from the above table caused by multiple factors. As mentioned above a two-hit or multiple -hit mechanism is thought to be the underlying pathomechanism, where the first hit is the increase of fat in the liver, followed by several additional factors that trigger inflammatory processes in the liver.

Table 1. Risk factors of NAFLD (table modified from [35]).

Modifiable factor	Non -modifiable factor
obesity	male gender
waist circumference >95th centile	roma origin
sedentary lifestyle	family history of NAFLD or T2DM
consumption of sugar/fructose sweetened beverages	parental (maternal) obesity
OSAS	ow birth weight
not breastfed	genetic diseases (Turner, Down sy, glycogenosis, *etc.*)

Insulin resistance has a close relationship with fatty liver, though it is not fully understood yet, whether insulin resistance triggers fat accumulation in the liver, or hepatic steatosis exacerbates insulin resistance. Extensive study is conducted to clarify this issue, though evidence is growing that NAFLD is an independent risk factor for atherosclerosis already in children regardless of insulin resistance.

The main environmental factor inducing accumulation of liver fat is the energy-dense, high fat, high fructose diet combined with sedentary lifestyle [35]. Energy intake at all ages was shown to be positively associated with most markers of NAFLD, except liver fibrosis [36].

Only a small percentage of patients progress from simple steatohepatosis to steatohepatitis. This is partly due to the amount of fat accumulated, the lipid profile, gut microbiota, genetic factors [28, 40].

DIAGNOSIS AND PROGNOSIS

On one hand there are no specific signs or symptoms associated with fatty liver in children but fatigability. On the other hand, obesity, OSAS syndrome, hypertension, hyperinsulinaemia, acanthosis nigricans are frequently observed symptoms. Visceral obesity is one of the major risk factors. Obesity (body mass index of greater than +2SD) is usually present. Not obesity per se, but BMI gain during childhood was proved to have strong correlation with adult NAFLD according to a longitudinal, large cohort examination [37].

In our department, we follow a group consisting of almost 300 overweighted and obese teenagers. 98% of them have alimentary obesity with associated complications like liver function alteration, insulin resistance, hyperinsulinaemia, acanthosis nigricans, sonographic alteration, elevated blood sugar, visceral fat accumulation.

Diagnosis of NAFLD is done by careful physical examination and screening in the absence of specific signs and symptoms. Nevertheless there are some nonspecific, but frequently observed symptoms, like hyperinsulinemia, hypertension, acanthosis nigricans, wheezing and sleep apnea. Obesity is a risk factor, especially visceral obesity. An increase in weight with 10% or more per year is likely to be present. That raises the importance of careful and detailed medical history, including family history in the evaluation. Children who have elevated transaminase levels should be even more carefully examined, primary infectious diseases, like hepatitis, viral hepatopathies (CMV, EBV infections) excluded. Some metabolic diseases (thyroid alterations, alfa-1-antitripsisn depletion, ceruloplasmin, ferritin alterations) should be ruled out.

In adolescents, nowadays alcohol history should be evaluated, as this can alter our diagnostic and therapeutic procedure:

- Clinical examination is based on physical examination, Anthropometric measurements (multifrequence bioimpedance measurement), waist circumference.
- Laboratory tests (liver function, lipid profile, high sensitivity CRP, blood glucose, insulin, *etc.*).
- Imaging modalities: sonography belongs to the first line examinations in the diagnosis of steatohepatitis, being non-invasive, unlimitedly repeatable, simple, cost-effective, so it is very convenient for the diagnosis and follow-up of children.

The principle of sonography (US): the presence of fat vacuoles within hepatocytes modifies the acoustic properties of the liver tissue. New methods are emerging, *e.g.*, transient and shear-wave elastography.

The sensitivity of US examinations increased in recent years due to technological advances, so diffuse, even and tightly packed echos are considered to be steatosis. Diagnosis is reliable in moderate to severe forms of the disease, but mild steatosis is difficult to be detected. In a recent prospective evaluation, US proved to have 90% sensitivity in detecting steatosis involving at least 20% of hepatocytes, but its sensitivity is lower when lower percent of cells are involved [38].

It is concluded in practice that a sonographic examination positive for steatosis means steatosis > 20% of hepatocytes, while negative sonography cannot exclude a lower amount of fat content. Nevertheless, US is used widely in the everyday settings in our hospital as well due to its simple, non-invasive procedure.

- Histological examination: in adults liver biopsy is performed being the gold-standard examination in the diagnosis and staging of NAFLD, but in pediatric population this relatively invasive procedure is seldomly used in the diagnosis of NAFLD being expensive, having the risk of complications.

Frequently, but not always, steatohepatosis can be detected by elevated transaminases and ultrasonographic alteration. At the same time, one has to keep in mind that normal liver function tests do not exclude NAFLD in children!

THERAPY AND FOLLOW-UP OF PATIENTS

The treatment of NAFLD in children differs greatly from that of adults. The primary goal is to treat the metabolic changes present.

In childhood, this means lifestyle modification. Weight loss (normalization) with dietary intervention and increased physical activity improves insulin sensitivity, and decreases tissue alterations. Nevertheless, quick weight loss might cause inflammation, fibrosis, so weight loss should be gradual, 0.5- 1kg/week. 7-10% weight loss might reduce liver steatosis by 40-50%. Daily physical activity for 30 minutes reduces insulin resistance, which is advantageous.

When designing food, the advantageous ones are those, which have a lower glycemic index, do not raise blood sugar and need no, or few insulin to metabolize.

In the past few years, surgical treatment has been used in childhood more frequently in morbidly obese persons, but this is not an everyday procedure.

In the past few years, some drugs are also used in children and adolescents to alter some pathologic conditions. Hypertension is most frequently treated with ACE inhibitor, or ARB blokker. Sometimes inhibition of lipase is used with ezetimibe administration.

In severe insulin resistance and liver function deterioration, insulin sensitizers can be used. Metformin is used in the United States for insulin resistance, it is not approved for that purpose in our country.

In our practice, lifestyle modification proved to be effective in the reversal of liver function tests and steatosis, though these parameters do not have close relationship with one another.

This multitask activity needs multidisciplinary team to support children and their caregivers. It is not enough to give advice about food to be taken and exercise to be done, but a continous motivation is needed to keep families on the track. Diabetologist or oncologist dietitian, physiotherapeutist, psychologist should be a part of the team.

CONCLUSION

NAFLD has emerged as the leading cause of chronic liver disease in children and adolescents causing severe metabolic alterations. A rapid rise in the rate of overweight and obese children over the last decade is most probably responsible for NAFLD epidemic. Emerging data suggest that although pathophysiology differs from adults, children with stetohepatitis also progresses to cirrhosis which increases liver-related morbidity and mortality.

There are different therapeutic approaches, but till now no evidence based intervention is available to improve liver damage because the disease has various causes, ranging from unhealthy diet to gut diseases and epigenetic factors.

Large scale, randomized-controlled trials are needed to define pharmacologic therapy in the pediatric population. Deeper understanding the underlying causes could help in the personalization of therapy.

Till then public health awareness and intervention are necessary to promote healthy lifestyle, *i.e.*, nutrition, exercise to reduce te burden of disease in the family and society.

CONFLICT OF INTEREST

The author confirms that author has no conflict of interest to declare for this publication.

ACKNOWLEDGEMENTS

Declared none.

REFERENCES

[1]   Sanders RH, Han A, Baker JS, Cobley S. Childhood obesity and its physical and psychological co-morbidities: a systematic review of Australian children and adolescents. Eur J Pediatr 2015; 174(6): 715-46.
        [http://dx.doi.org/10.1007/s00431-015-2551-3] [PMID: 25922141]

[2]   Feldstein AE, Charatcharoenwitthaya P, Treeprasertsuk S, Benson JT, Enders FB, Angulo P. The natural history of non-alcoholic fatty liver disease in children: a follow-up study for up to 20 years. Gut 2009; 58(11): 1538-44.
        [http://dx.doi.org/10.1136/gut.2008.171280] [PMID: 19625277]

[3]   Patton HM, Sirlin C, Behling C, Middleton M, Schwimmer JB, Lavine JE. Pediatric nonalcoholic fatty liver disease: a critical appraisal of current data and implications for future research. J Pediatr Gastroenterol Nutr 2006; 43(4): 413-27.
        [http://dx.doi.org/10.1097/01.mpg.0000239995.58388.56] [PMID: 17033514]

[4]   Nobili V, Alkhouri N, Alisi A, *et al.* Nonalcoholic fatty liver disease: a challenge for pediatricians. JAMA Pediatr 2015; 169(2): 170-6.
        [http://dx.doi.org/10.1001/jamapediatrics.2014.2702] [PMID: 25506780]

[5]   Ortiz-Lopez C, Lomonaco R, Orsak B, *et al.* Prevalence of prediabetes and diabetes and metabolic profile of patients with nonalcoholic fatty liver disease (NAFLD). Diabetes Care 2012; 35(4): 873-8.
        [http://dx.doi.org/10.2337/dc11-1849] [PMID: 22374640]

[6]   Weiß J, Rau M, Geier A. Non-alcoholic fatty liver disease: epidemiology, clinical course, investigation, and treatment. Dtsch Arztebl Int 2014; 111(26): 447-52.
        [PMID: 25019921]

[7]   Vernon G, Baranova A, Younossi ZM. Systematic review: the epidemiology and natural history of non-alcoholic fatty liver disease and non-alcoholic steatohepatitis in adults. Aliment Pharmacol Ther 2011; 34(3): 274-85.
        [http://dx.doi.org/10.1111/j.1365-2036.2011.04724.x] [PMID: 21623852]

[8]   Leite NC, Salles GF, Araujo AL, Villela-Nogueira CA, Cardoso CR. Prevalence and associated factors of non-alcoholic fatty liver disease in patients with type-2 diabetes mellitus. Liver Int 2009; 29(1): 113-9.
        [http://dx.doi.org/10.1111/j.1478-3231.2008.01718.x] [PMID: 18384521]

[9]   Peeters A, Barendregt JJ, Willekens F, Mackenbach JP, Al Mamun A, Bonneux L. Obesity in adulthood and its consequences for life expectancy: a life-table analysis. Ann Intern Med 2003; 138(1): 24-32.
        [http://dx.doi.org/10.7326/0003-4819-138-1-200301070-00008] [PMID: 12513041]

[10]   DAdamo E, Cali AM, Weiss R, *et al.* Central role of fatty liver in the pathogenesis of insulin resistance in obese adolescents. Diabetes Care 2010; 33(8): 1817-22.
        [http://dx.doi.org/10.2337/dc10-0284] [PMID: 20668154]

[11]   Denzer C, Thiere D, Muche R, *et al.* Gender-specific prevalences of fatty liver in obese children and adolescents: roles of body fat distribution, sex steroids, and insulin resistance. J Clin Endocrinol Metab 2009; 94(10): 3872-81.
        [http://dx.doi.org/10.1210/jc.2009-1125] [PMID: 19773396]

[12]   Adams LA, Lymp JF, St Sauver J, *et al.* The natural history of nonalcoholic fatty liver disease: a population-based cohort study. Gastroenterology 2005; 129(1): 113-21.
[http://dx.doi.org/10.1053/j.gastro.2005.04.014] [PMID: 16012941]

[13]   Kasturiratne A, Weerasinghe S, Dassanayake AS, *et al.* Influence of non-alcoholic fatty liver disease on the development of diabetes mellitus. J Gastroenterol Hepatol 2013; 28(1): 142-7.
[http://dx.doi.org/10.1111/j.1440-1746.2012.07264.x] [PMID: 22989165]

[14]   Zelber-Sagi S, Lotan R, Shibolet O, *et al.* Non-alcoholic fatty liver disease independently predicts prediabetes during a 7-year prospective follow-up. Liver Int 2013; 33(9): 1406-12.
[http://dx.doi.org/10.1111/liv.12200] [PMID: 23656177]

[15]   Swinburn BA, Sacks G, Hall KD, *et al.* The global obesity pandemic: shaped by global drivers and local environments. Lancet 2011; 378(9793): 804-14.
[http://dx.doi.org/10.1016/S0140-6736(11)60813-1] [PMID: 21872749]

[16]   Feldstein AE, Charatcharoenwitthaya P, Treeprasertsuk S, Benson JT, Enders FB, Angulo P. The natural history of non-alcoholic fatty liver disease in children: a follow-up study for up to 20 years. Gut 2009; 58(11): 1538-44.
[http://dx.doi.org/10.1136/gut.2008.171280] [PMID: 19625277]

[17]   Nobili V. Non-alcoholic fatty liver disease in children and adolescents. Clin Biochem 2014; 47(9): 720.
[http://dx.doi.org/10.1016/j.clinbiochem.2014.05.025] [PMID: 24854694]

[18]   Marzuillo P, Del Giudice EM, Santoro N. Pediatric non-alcoholic fatty liver disease: New insights and future directions. World J Hepatol 2014; 6(4): 217-25.
[http://dx.doi.org/10.4254/wjh.v6.i4.217] [PMID: 24799990]

[19]   Brumbaugh DE, Friedman JE. Developmental origins of nonalcoholic fatty liver disease. Pediatr Res 2014; 75(1-2): 140-7.
[http://dx.doi.org/10.1038/pr.2013.193] [PMID: 24192698]

[20]   Angulo P. Nonalcoholic fatty liver disease. N Engl J Med 2002; 346(16): 1221-31.
[http://dx.doi.org/10.1056/NEJMra011775] [PMID: 11961152]

[21]   Tie HT, Xia YY, Zeng YS, *et al.* Risk of childhood overweight or obesity associated with excessive weight gain during pregnancy: a meta-analysis. Arch Gynecol Obstet 2014; 289(2): 247-57.
[http://dx.doi.org/10.1007/s00404-013-3053-z] [PMID: 24141389]

[22]   Patro B, Liber A, Zalewski B, Poston L, Szajewska H, Koletzko B. Maternal and paternal body mass index and offspring obesity: a systematic review. Ann Nutr Metab 2013; 63(1-2): 32-41.
[http://dx.doi.org/10.1159/000350313] [PMID: 23887153]

[23]   Arata M, Nakajima J, Nishimata S, Nagata T, Kawashima H. Nonalcoholic steatohepatitis and insulin resistance in children. World J Diabetes 2014; 5(6): 917-23.
[http://dx.doi.org/10.4239/wjd.v5.i6.917] [PMID: 25512797]

[24]   Tamura S, Shimomura I. Contribution of adipose tissue and de novo lipogenesis to nonalcoholic fatty liver disease. J Clin Invest 2005; 115(5): 1139-42.
[http://dx.doi.org/10.1172/JCI24930] [PMID: 15864343]

[25]   Moran JR, Ghishan FK, Halter SA, Greene HL. Steatohepatitis in obese children: a cause of chronic liver dysfunction. Am J Gastroenterol 1983; 78(6): 374-7.
[PMID: 6859017]

[26]   Pacifico L, Cantisani V, Ricci P, *et al.* Nonalcoholic fatty liver disease and carotid atherosclerosis in children. Pediatr Res 2008; 63(4): 423-7.
[http://dx.doi.org/10.1203/PDR.0b013e318165b8e7] [PMID: 18356751]

[27] Demircioğlu F, Koçyiğit A, Arslan N, Cakmakçi H, Hizli S, Sedat AT. Intima-media thickness of carotid artery and susceptibility to atherosclerosis in obese children with nonalcoholic fatty liver disease. J Pediatr Gastroenterol Nutr 2008; 47(1): 68-75.
[http://dx.doi.org/10.1097/MPG.0b013e31816232c9] [PMID: 18607271]

[28] Jin R, Le NA, Cleeton R, *et al.* Amount of hepatic fat predicts cardiovascular risk independent of insulin resistance among Hispanic-American adolescents. Lipids Health Dis 2015; 14: 39.
[http://dx.doi.org/10.1186/s12944-015-0038-x] [PMID: 25925168]

[29] Packard CJ. Small dense low-density lipoprotein and its role as an independent predictor of cardiovascular disease. Curr Opin Lipidol 2006; 17(4): 412-7.
[http://dx.doi.org/10.1097/01.mol.0000236367.42755.c1] [PMID: 16832165]

[30] Rizzo M, Berneis K. Small, dense low-density-lipoproteins and the metabolic syndrome. Diabetes Metab Res Rev 2007; 23(1): 14-20.
[http://dx.doi.org/10.1002/dmrr.694] [PMID: 17080469]

[31] Birkenfeld AL, Shulman GI. Nonalcoholic fatty liver disease, hepatic insulin resistance, and type 2 diabetes. Hepatology 2014; 59(2): 713-23.
[http://dx.doi.org/10.1002/hep.26672] [PMID: 23929732]

[32] Jornayvaz FR, Shulman GI. Diacylglycerol activation of protein kinase Cε and hepatic insulin resistance. Cell Metab 2012; 15(5): 574-84.
[http://dx.doi.org/10.1016/j.cmet.2012.03.005] [PMID: 22560210]

[33] DeFilippis AP, Blaha MJ, Martin SS, *et al.* Nonalcoholic fatty liver disease and serum lipoproteins: the Multi-Ethnic Study of Atherosclerosis. Atherosclerosis 2013; 227(2): 429-36.
[http://dx.doi.org/10.1016/j.atherosclerosis.2013.01.022] [PMID: 23419204]

[34] Schwimmer JB, Behling C, Newbury R, *et al.* Histopathology of pediatric nonalcoholic fatty liver disease. Hepatology 2005; 42(3): 641-9.
[http://dx.doi.org/10.1002/hep.20842] [PMID: 16116629]

[35] Mann JP, Goonetilleke R, McKiernan P. Paediatric non-alcoholic fatty liver disease: a practical overview for non-specialists. Arch Dis Child 2015; 100(7): 673-7.
[http://dx.doi.org/10.1136/archdischild-2014-307985] [PMID: 25633064]

[36] Anderson EL, Howe LD, Fraser A, *et al.* Childhood energy intake is associated with nonalcoholic fatty liver disease in adolescents. J Nutr 2015; 145(5): 983-9.
[http://dx.doi.org/10.3945/jn.114.208397] [PMID: 25788585]

[37] Zimmermann E, Gamborg M, Holst C, Baker JL, Sørensen TI, Berentzen TL. Body mass index in school-aged children and the risk of routinely diagnosed non-alcoholic fatty liver disease in adulthood: a prospective study based on the Copenhagen School Health Records Register. BMJ Open 2015; 5(4): e006998.
[http://dx.doi.org/10.1136/bmjopen-2014-006998] [PMID: 25941179]

[38] Strauss S, Gavish E, Gottlieb P, Katsnelson L. Interobserver and intraobserver variability in the sonographic assessment of fatty liver. AJR Am J Roentgenol 2007; 189(6): W320-3.
[http://dx.doi.org/10.2214/AJR.07.2123] [PMID: 18029843]

[39] Widhalm K, Ghods E. Nonalcoholic fatty liver disease: a challenge for pediatricians. Int J Obes 2010; 34(10): 1451-67.
[http://dx.doi.org/10.1038/ijo.2010.185] [PMID: 20838401]

[40] Paolella G, Mandato C, Pierri L, Poeta M, Di Stasi M, Vajro P. Gut-liver axis and probiotics: their role in non-alcoholic fatty liver disease. World J Gastroenterol 2014; 20(42): 15518-31.
[http://dx.doi.org/10.3748/wjg.v20.i42.15518] [PMID: 25400436]

SUBJECT INDEX

A
Adipose expansion 137, 142

C
Cancer prevention 134, 137, 139, 148, 150
Cancer surveillance 137, 148, 151
Cardiovascular diseases ii, 21, 23, 47, 52, 103, 111, 164
Cardiovascular risk 13, 32, 72, 112, 164, 169, 176
Children i, iii, 25, 26, 34, 47, 52, 57, 60, 69, 75, 119, 129, 162, 164-176
Cholesterol 8, 22, 53, 80, 83, 88, 96, 103, 114, 126, 127, 145, 159, 169
Cirrhosis i, 16, 17, 39, 42, 46, 47, 50, 51, 56, 57, 63, 64, 66, 70, 72, 74, 75, 77, 92, 94, 110, 119, 127, 134, 144, 146, 147, 158, 160, 161, 166, 173
Colorectal cancer 21, 27
Cryptogenic cirrhosis 7, 16, 17, 20, 63, 72, 74, 127, 134, 137, 142, 147, 160, 161

D
Diabetes i, ii, 3, 4, 16, 18, 29, 32, 33, 44, 47, 52, 57, 63, 68, 74, 78, 96, 103, 104, 106, 117, 125, 127, 133, 144, 148, 149, 151, 153, 157, 174-176
Dipeptidyl peptidase inhibitors 119
Dysbiosis 137, 145, 167
Dyslipidemia ii, 12, 13, 63, 103, 104, 108, 111, 115, 116, 125, 150

E
Epidemiology i, 7, 13, 15, 16, 19, 72, 111, 112, 130, 138, 151, 165, 174

F
Fat suppression 36
Fibroscan 36, 38, 39

H
Hepatocarcinogenesis 137, 150, 151, 153, 154, 156, 158, 159
Hepatocellular carcinoma i, 8, 16, 19, 20, 27, 36, 37, 46, 47, 74, 75, 77, 96, 120, 130, 137, 138, 158-163
HOMA-IR 103, 105
Hyperinsulinemia 73, 85, 114, 137, 144, 149, 169, 171
Hyperlipidemia 12, 110, 119-121
Hypertension ii, 3, 10, 21, 22, 47, 57, 103, 104, 116, 120, 138, 148, 171, 172

I
Incretins 119
Inflammation 10, 21, 22, 28, 29, 40, 46, 52, 53, 60, 73, 77, 78, 80, 92, 95, 103, 105, 107, 112, 114, 116, 119, 120, 122, 129, 131, 143, 150, 156, 158, 166, 167, 172
Insulin resistance i, ii, 3, 5, 16, 21, 22, 24, 27, 32, 47, 53, 63, 64, 70, 72, 73, 81, 83, 84, 94, 96, 97, 99, 103, 105, 106, 108, 131, 137, 144, 150, 169-176

L
Lifestyle modification i, 11, 119, 131, 164, 172, 173
Lipid disorder 103
Lipotoxicity 52, 53, 61, 72, 74, 77, 85, 87, 90, 91, 94, 99, 112, 121, 137, 143, 144
Liver Biopsy 3, 5, 6, 9, 14, 15, 21, 28, 31, 36, 47, 56, 63, 65, 67, 71, 72, 76, 107, 110, 140, 153, 172
Liver CT liver imaging 36
Liver MRI 36
Liver ultrasound 36

Tatjana Ábel & Gabriella Lengyel (Eds.)
All rights reserved-© 2017 Bentham Science Publishers

www.ingramcontent.com/pod-product-compliance
Lightning Source LLC
Chambersburg PA
CBHW041728210326
41598CB00008B/808